TEACHINGS OF YOGA

TEACHINGS
OF YOGA

EDITED BY

Georg Feuerstein

SHAMBHALA
Boston & London
1997

DEDICATED TO
YOGA MASTERS & PRACTITIONERS
EVERYWHERE

Shambhala Publications, Inc.
Horticultural Hall
300 Massachusetts Avenue
Boston, Massachusetts 02115
www.shambhala.com

9 8 7 6 5 4 3 2

Printed in Canada

Book design and composition by Wesley B. Tanner/Passim Editions

⊖ This edition is printed on acid-free paper that meets
the American National Standards Institute Z39.48 Standard.

Distributed in the United States by Random House, Inc.,
and in Canada by Random House of Canada Ltd

LIBRARY OF CONGRESS CATALOGING-IN-PUBLICATION DATA

Teachings of yoga/edited by Georg Feuerstein.—1st ed.
   p.   cm.
   Includes bibliographical references.
   ISBN 1-57062-318-X (pbk.:alk. paper)
   1. Yoga.   I. Feuerstein, Georg.
B132.Y6Y43   1997
181'.45—dc21
                                               97-7507
                                               CIP

Yoga Is the Greatest Virtue

Verily, there is no virtue greater than Yoga,
no good greater than Yoga,
and no subtlety greater than Yoga.
There is nothing that is greater than Yoga.

YOGA-SHIKHĀ-UPANISHAD

Contents

Editor's Preface

Four thousand or more years ago, Prince Arjuna found himself embroiled in one of the fiercest wars ever fought on Indian soil. On the morning of the first of eighteen battles, he was shaken by the recognition that he would have to fight and possibly maim or even kill his kinsmen and former teachers among the ranks of the enemy. He was confused and on the verge of abdicating his responsibilities as a military leader when the god-man Krishna intervened. He, an incarnation of the Divine itself, instructed the perplexed prince in the necessity of fighting for what is true and lawful (*dharma*) and sparing no effort to conquer the forces of evil. Krishna taught that to make sense of the seemingly senseless task confronting Arjuna, the prince must remove his vision from the material realm and open his eyes to the spiritual reality, the Divine Being. Then everything would fall into place, ending the confusion. Having been thus instructed, Arjuna realized that he must not succumb to inaction out of fear but make a conscious choice. He opted to fight, yet to do so without self-interest, hatred, or resentment — the great ideal of *karma-yoga*, the path of self-transcending action.

The classic dialogue between Arjuna and Krishna, as captured for posterity in the famous *Bhagavad-Gītā* ("Lord's Song"), undoubtedly has historical roots. But its abiding significance is as an allegory of spiritual life, which always demands that we untiringly confront the darkness of egoism, of demerit, within ourselves. Arjuna typifies the spiritual seeker who, until he has received illumining instruction from a qualified teacher, walks through life in ignorance, causing himself and others much needless suffering. Krishna is the enlightened being, who simply goes with the flow of life. As he points out to his royal disciple, he is Arjuna's own innermost Self.

All of us have a Krishna and an Arjuna component in our nature. We are both Self (or Spirit) and self (or ego-bound personality). To the degree that we can transcend or, as the Sanskrit scriptures say, "conquer" the self, we increasingly realize — that is, become present *as* — our true Self. According to the testimony of the great sages, this Self is immortal, omniscient, omnipresent, luminous, blissful, and forever free from all ill. It can never be lost, but we must rediscover it by cleansing the mirror of our own mind. The mind is the alchemical mercury that must be transmuted into pure gold. It is also the cauldron in which this process of transformation occurs. The yogis are great spiritual alchemists whose secret work is their own metamorphosis.

All of us are at least potentially capable of the same work. Sooner or later, when we have understood enough about human existence, we are challenged to undertake it. Some will advance quickly on the path, others more slowly. But, as the *Bhagavad-Gītā* (2.40) assures us, no effort is ever lost. We do, however, need to take the first step, and then the next and the next. If we apply ourselves consistently and with faith to this self-transformative path, we will succeed and attain enlightenment. This is the central message of all forms of Yoga, be it *karma-yoga* (the path of self-transcending action), *bhakti-yoga* (the path of self-transcending love-devotion), *jnāna-yoga* (the path of wisdom), *rāja-yoga* (the royal path of meditation), *hatha-yoga* (the forceful path of bodily transformation), *mantra-yoga* (the path of numinous sound), *tāraka-yoga* (the path of light), *tantra-yoga* (the path of ecstatic realization), or *sahaja-yoga* (the path of spontaneity).

Enlightenment means recovering our true identity as the Self, or Spirit. This magnificent inner event spells the end of all our suffering and confusion. It means coming home.

What then? Westerners, who tend to be fond of action, are troubled by the prospect of eternal lotus eating. But enlightenment contains no prescription for living. Among the greatest adepts of India have been cave-dwelling eremites as well as kings. As the *Bhagavad-Gītā* (2.48) states: "Yoga is said to be equanimity." The Sanskrit term *samatva*, usually rendered as "equanimity," means literally "sameness," and here refers to the accomplished yogi's superb ability to see the same —

the Same One — in everyone and everything. Whether adepts are active or passive is irrelevant and merely a matter of personal inclination or innate nature (*svabhāva*). When they do act, however, they invariably demonstrate skill. Hence the *Bhagavad-Gītā* (2.50) appropriately defines Yoga as "skill in action." Enlightenment brings sublime ease to the business of living. By removing the illusion of the ego, it eradicates suffering, though not the challenges of finite existence, including illness and loss.

The word *yoga*, as has often been pointed out, means "union" and also "discipline." Addressing the former connotation, the elephant-shaped god Ganesha explains in the *Ganesha-Gītā* (1.6–9, 20b):

Sages do not say, "Yoga is union." Yoga is not union with wealth. Yoga is not union with objects or the elements.

O King of men, Yoga is not union with fathers, mothers, and others; or union with kinsfolk, sons, and others; or union with the eight supernatural powers.

All this is not Yoga. Yoga is not union with a woman who, in this world, has a beautiful body, or union with sovereignty. Nor is it union with elephants and horses.

Yoga is not even union with Indra's realm, so agreeable to Yoga aspirants. I maintain that Yoga is not union with the abode of truth either.

> . . . I affirm that the Yoga consisting in the attitude of
> nonseparation is the perfect Yoga.

That is to say, the great adepts unite themselves only
with the ultimate Self, which is the same in all beings.
Viewing everything from this vantage point, they make
no absolute distinctions, whether they choose to be
active or immersed in contemplation. This is the acme
of the unitive discipline called Yoga.

Most Yoga scriptures are fairly technical and some
are even extremely technical, brimming with
difficult philosophical and metaphysical notions, as
well as recondite descriptions of advanced spiritual
practices. To compile an anthology that will be helpful
to beginners, I have scanned numerous texts originally
composed in Sanskrit, Hindi, Marathi, and Tamil to
identify those passages that in themselves are characteristic of the yogic approach yet are not burdened with
overly difficult concepts or practices that would mean
little to the neophyte Western seeker without lengthy
explanations or tedious footnotes.

The purpose of this anthology, after all, is primarily
to edify and only secondarily to instruct, while at the
same time preserving the integrity of the Yoga tradition.
The quotations in this volume were chosen for their
inspirational power. They still speak to us across the
centuries because the human condition has remained
essentially the same throughout history: We either are
free from the clutches of the ego personality (*ahamkāra*)

or are bound by it. We either live as the Self, which is the same in all beings, or experience ourselves as separate islands. We either are blissful or are hunting whatever temporary pleasures we can get because we are basically suffering. We either are a compassionate presence in the world or are engaged in the struggle for survival, which inevitably leads us to harm others. We either *are* love or constantly look to be loved. We either *are* present as the Self or habitually dramatize the illusory ego self.

Remember, most of the selections stem from texts that were composed or originally spoken by qualified adepts in the art and science of Yoga, masters of the senses and the mind, whose vision penetrated deep into the mysteries of existence. Because their wisdom is timeless, we can benefit from it as much as did the spiritual seekers of yore. I have also included excerpts from the writings or sayings of more recent masters, such as Sri Ramakrishna, Swami Vivekananda, Swami Sivananda, Sri Aurobindo, Swami Rama Tirtha, Meher Baba, "Mahatma" Gandhi, Paramahamsa Yogananda, Swami Muktananda, Nisargadatta Maharaj, Gopi Krishna, and Swami Sivananda Radha. However, tempted as I was, I have refrained from dipping into the works of still living authorities of Yoga, mainly to avoid giving the impression of partiality.

The quotes have been loosely arranged to proceed from a consideration of the nature of human existence and embodiment to the need for renunciation and mind training, to an explanation of discipleship and initiation through a qualified teacher, to an outline of the yogic path itself, ending with higher states of consciousness and liberation, including several ecstatic utterances by great adepts.

The tradition of Yoga spans not only more than four thousand years but also many Indic schools of thought and has proven influential in the development of Hinduism, Buddhism, Jainism, and Sikhism. The focus of the present anthology is exclusively on Hindu Yoga in its preclassical, classical, and postclassical manifestations. I have written at length about the seminal aspects of the various phases of the Yoga tradition in my other books. Here I am baring the very heart of Yoga. I believe that by carefully reading and pondering the selections in this little volume, you will not only come to a real understanding of the essential teachings of Yoga but also be pulled into their field of resonance. In this way, your own spiritual life will be greatly enriched.

Listening (*shravana*) to the disclosures of sages and saints is one of the time-honored practices of seekers after the Truth. Any time we pay attention to anything, we participate in it on the subtle levels. Therefore it matters greatly where we place our attention. The sages long ago recommended that the next best thing to immersing oneself in the Truth directly through profound meditation and ecstasy is to hear it from the mouth of one who knows and then to ponder it with one's native reasoning ability.

Let us, then, listen well that we might benefit from the communications of the illustrious finders of Truth, the Self-realized masters of the distant and the more recent past.

On the Way to the Divine

The ascent to the divine Life is the human journey, the Work of works, the acceptable Sacrifice. This alone is man's real business in the world and the justification of his existence, without which he would be only an insect crawling among other ephemeral insects on a speck of surface mud and water which has managed to form itself amid the appalling immensities of the physical universe.

SRI AUROBINDO

This excerpt, like almost all the other excerpts in this anthology, was composed long before feminism made us aware of the gender bias in our language. Like English, Sanskrit employs masculine pronouns for generic statements. The editor asks his readers to kindly bear this fact in mind.

The Preciousness of
Human Embodiment

Lord Shiva said:

After obtaining a human body, which is difficult to obtain and which serves as a ladder to liberation, who is more sinful than he who does not cross over to the Self?

Therefore, upon obtaining the best possible life form, he who does not know his own good is merely killing himself.

How can one come to know the purpose of human life without a human body? Hence, having obtained the gift of a human body, one should perform meritorious deeds.

One should completely protect oneself by oneself. Oneself is the vessel for everything. One should make an effort in protecting oneself. Otherwise the Truth cannot be seen.

Village, house, land, money, even auspicious and inauspicious karma can be obtained over and over again, but not a human body.

People always make an effort to protect the body. They do not wish to abandon the body even when sick with leprosy and other diseases.

For the purpose of attaining knowledge, the virtuous person should preserve the body with effort. Knowledge aims at the Yoga of meditation. He will be liberated quickly.

If one does not guard oneself against that which is inauspicious, then who, intent on the good, will ever cross over to the Self?

He who does not heal himself from hellish diseases while here on Earth, what can he do about his disease when he goes to a place where no remedy exists?

What fool starts digging a well when his house is already on fire? So long as this body exists, one should cultivate the Truth.

Old age is like a tigress; life runs out like water in a broken pot; diseases strike like enemies. Therefore one should cultivate the highest good now.

One should cultivate the highest good while the senses are not yet frail, suffering is not yet firmly rooted, and adversities have not yet become overwhelming.

Kula-Arnava-Tantra

The Time to Realize God Is Now

We do not obtain a human life
Just for the asking.
Birth in a human body
Is the reward for good deeds
Done in former lives.
Life waxes and wanes imperceptibly,
And it does not last long.
Once fallen, a leaf
Does not return to the branch.
Behold the ocean of cyclic existence,
With its swift, irresistible tide.
O beloved Lord, pilot of my soul,
Swiftly conduct my barque to the farther shore.
Mira is the slave of the beloved Lord.
She says: Life lasts but a few days.

MĪRĀBĀĪ

The Significance of Human Life

❀

Sage Prahlāda said:

When still young, the wise person should cultivate the virtues dear to the Divine. A human birth is difficult to obtain here on Earth, and even though human life is fleeting, it is full of significance.

Thus one should approach the Lord's feet, for He is the good-hearted ruler of the self of all creatures and is dear to them.

Sensory pleasures, like pain, are harvested effortlessly by embodied beings everywhere, simply on account of their destiny.

One should make no effort to obtain pleasure, for that would be a waste of life and would not bring the supreme peace that springs alone from the Lord's lotus feet.

Therefore an intelligent person who is caught up in the world should struggle for peace while the human body is still flourishing rather than failing.

The span of human life is a hundred years. Half of this is wasted by a person lacking self-control, because he sleeps stuporously in the dark of night.

Twenty years go by in childhood, when one is bewildered, and in youth, when one is preoccupied with playing; another twenty years go by in old age, when one is physically impaired and lacking in determination.

The remaining years are wasted by that person who, out of great confusion and insatiable desire, is madly attached to family life.

How can a person who is attached to family life, with his senses uncontrolled and bound by strong ties of affection, liberate himself?

Bhāgavata-Purāna

The Potential of the Body

Sage Vasishtha said:

For the ignorant person, this body is the source of endless suffering; but to the wise person, this body is the source of infinite delight.

For the wise person, its loss is no loss at all, but while it persists it is completely a source of delight for the wise person.

For the wise person, the body serves as a vehicle that can transport him swiftly in this world and is known as a chariot for attaining liberation and unending enjoyment.

Since the body affords the wise person the experience of sound, sight, taste, touch, and smell as well as prosperity and friendship, it brings him gain.

Even though the body exposes one to a whole string of painful and joyous activities, the omniscient sage can patiently bear all experiences.

The wise person reigns, free from feverish unhappiness, over the city known as the body, even as Vāsava [Indra] dwells in his city free from distress.

It does not cast him into the pit of pride like a high-mettled horse, nor does it cause him to abandon his "daughter" of wisdom to evil greed and so forth.

Yoga-Vāsishtha

Strengthen the Body to Liberate the Mind

❀

Sage Gheranda said:

There is no fetter like illusion (*māyā*); there is no power greater than Yoga; there is no friend better than wisdom and no enemy worse than the ego (*ahamkāra*).

Just as one learns the sciences by first practicing the alphabet, so one attains the knowledge of Truth by cultivating Yoga.

The body of creatures arises from their good or bad deeds. In turn, the body causes karma, and thus the waterwheel of existence revolves.

Just as the waterwheel revolves by the strength of bullocks, so the individual revolves through life and death by the force of karma.

The body always wears away like an unbaked clay pot placed in water. Therefore one should cultivate bodily fitness by tempering it with the fire of Yoga.

Gheranda-Samhitā

Microcosm and Macrocosm

Within this body exist Mount Meru, the seven continents, lakes, oceans, mountains, plains, and the protectors of these plains.

In it also dwell the seers, the sages, all the stars and planets, the sacred river crossings and pilgrimage centers, and the deities of these centers.

In it whirl the sun and the moon, which are the causes of creation and annihilation. Likewise, it contains ether, air, fire, water, and earth.

All beings embodied in the three worlds, which are connected to Mount Meru, exist in the body together with all their activities.

He who knows all this is a yogi. There is no doubt about this.

Shiva-Samhitā

The Transmuted Body of the Yogi

❀

Everyone is conquered by the body. But the yogis conquer the body. Hence how can the fruit of karma, such as pleasure and pain, affect them?

He who has conquered the senses, the mind, the higher mind (*buddhi*), desire, anger, and so forth, has conquered all. By what could he possibly be disturbed?

As the great elements and the other principles of existence are gradually involuted, the body made from seven constituents is slowly consumed by the fire of Yoga.

Even the deities cannot see the immensely powerful yogic body, which is supreme, released from the bond of differentation, and endowed with various capacities.

This body is like space, even purer than space, more subtle than the subtle, appearing coarse yet not coarse, insentient yet sentient.

The master yogi, who is independent, can assume any form at will, and is beyond birth and death, sports anywhere in the three realms according to his play.

Such a yogi, who has mastered the senses and possesses incomprehensible powers, assumes diverse forms and then dissolves them again at will.

Through the power of Yoga, he is not subject to death. He has already died through *hatha-yoga*. How can death strike one already dead?

Where others are dead, there he is fully alive. But where ignorant people are alive, there he is surely dead.

There is nothing left for him to do, nor is he affected by what he does. Having become liberated in life, he is always transparent, free from every blemish.

Yoga-Shikhā-Upanishad

"I Am the Body" Is a Lie

The notion that I am the body is known as the "inner instrument."

The notion that I am the body is called the great cycle of existence.
The notion that I am the body is called bondage.

The notion that I am the body is called suffering.
The idea that I am the body is known as hell.

The notion that I am the body is said to be the whole world.
The notion that I am the body is described as the knot of the heart.

The idea that I am the body is called ignorance.
The idea that I am the body is verily the state of unreality.

The thought that I am the body is termed nescience.
The idea that I am the body is called duality.

The notion that I am the body is really the individual.
The idea that I am the body is described as that which is
limited.

The notion that I am the body is revealed to be the
great evil.
The thought that I am the body is certainly blemished
desire.
Even some notion of this is said to be the threefold
affliction.

Desire, anger, bondage are all suffering. The world,
which assumes various forms through time, is
blemished.
Whatever belongs to this whole web of notions, O
Somya, know that to be of the mind.

Tejo-Bindu-Upanishad

Fell the Tree of "I" and "Mine"

✿

"I" is the germination of the sprout; "mine" is a big tree trunk; home and land are its branches; children and wife are its shoots.

Wealth and gain are its big leaves. It grows more than once, and merit and demerit are its blossoms and joy and sorrow its fruit.

It overshadows the path to liberation, is watered by the sexual contact between fools, and is infested with the bees of desire. Lack of understanding about what should be done is the tree itself.

Those who are tired of the ways of the world and seek refuge under its shade become dependent on pleasure derived from false knowledge. How can they reach the end?

But those who fell the tree of "mineness" with the axe of wisdom, sharpened on the whetstone of association with the virtuous, travel along the right path.

Reaching the Absolute's cool grove, which is free from dirt and thorns, the wise who abstain from action attain the Supreme.

Mārkandeya-Purāna

The World Is Illusory

Lord Shiva said:

Just as a single form is imagined variously in dreams but upon waking is single again, so the world appears manifold as well.

Just as a rope is misperceived as a snake or mother-of-pearl is misperceived as silver, so the supreme Self is converted into this universe.

Just as the mistaken notion of a snake is removed by the recognition that it is a rope, so the mistaken idea of this world is corrected by the knowledge of the Self.

Just as the misperception of silver is corrected through the recognition that it is mother-of-pearl, likewise the misperception of the world is always corrected through knowledge of the Self.

The yogi who has renounced all conceptualization, upon abandoning his hold on the false reality, certainly perceives the Self by the Self in the Self.

Perceiving the Self, which is infinite and of the nature of happiness, by the Self in the Self, and forgetting the world, he delights in intense ecstasy (*samādhi*).

Shiva-Samhitā

The Fishing-Net of the World

🦚

This world is like a fishing-net. Men are the fish, and God, whose maya has created this world, is the fisherman. When the fish are entangled in the net, some of them try to tear through its meshes in order to get their liberation. They are like the men striving after liberation. But by no means all of them escape. Only a few jump out of the net with a loud splash, and then people say, "Ah! There goes a big one!" In like manner, three or four men attain liberation. Again, some fish are so careful by nature that they are never caught in the net; some beings of the ever-perfect class, like Narada, are never entangled in the meshes of worldliness. Most of the fish are trapped, but they are not conscious of the net and of their imminent death. No sooner are they entangled than they run headlong, net and all, trying to hide themselves in the mud. They don't make the least effort to get free. On the contrary, they go deeper and deeper into the mud. These fish are like the bound men. They are still inside the net, but they think they are quite safe there.

SRI RAMAKRISHNA

The Umbrella of Mental Impressions

In actuality, God is not far from the seeker, nor is it impossible to see Him. He is like the sun, which is ever shining right above you. It is you who have held over your head the umbrella of your variegated mental impressions which hide Him from your view. You have only to remove the umbrella and the Sun is there for you to see. It does not have to be brought there from anywhere. But such a tiny and trivial thing as an umbrella can deprive you of the sight of such a stupendous fact as the Sun.

MEHER BABA

Suffering Is Omnipresent

On reflection, there is always only suffering in all
the worlds, at the beginning, in the middle, and in
the end.

Sorrows are in the present and likewise in the future,
and there are manifold sorrows in places tainted by
faults.

Those who mistake ignorance for knowledge fail to
consider past sorrows. . . .

There is undoubtedly only suffering, yet the unin-
formed do not know this. O best of sages, this is so
even in the heavens, owing to the removal of impurities
and so forth.

Those who are seized by the various kinds of "illnesses," such as attachment, hatred, and fear, are like a
tree that inevitably falls to the ground when its roots
are cut.

Even the heaven dwellers tumble down to Earth when the tree of merit is destroyed. Those addicted to desiring sorrow will gain the experience of sorrow.

Linga-Purāna

The Truth about Joy and Sorrow

Suffering arises from the disease of desire. From the disease of sorrow arises joy. From joy springs sorrow, and thus it is over and over again. Sorrow is preceded by joy; joy is preceded by suffering.

When you experience sorrow after pleasure, you will again experience pleasure. Sorrow is not experienced forever, nor is pleasure experienced forever.

There is no friend like joy, and no enemy like sorrow. Wealth is not enough for the joyous, and wisdom is not enough for the wealthy.

Understanding does not lead to wealth. Stupidity does not lead to poverty. The wise person knows about the repetitive course of the world.

Joy comes to him who is entitled to it, whether he is wise, foolish, heroic, fearful, dull, intelligent, weak, or strong.

Those who are complete fools in the world and those who have attained the Supreme through understanding are people for whom joy flourishes. The person in between is troubled.

Mahābhārata

Cutting through Desire

In stone houses and stately halls, He is not.
In splendid parlors and massive temples, He is not.
In holy garbs, He is not.
But He is in the thoughts of those
who have overcome their desires.
Even though they have bodies of flesh,
He grants them liberation.

Sunder your desires! Sunder your desires!
Sunder your desires even unto the Lord!
The more your desires, the greater your sorrows.
The more you give up, the greater shall be your bliss.

Burn up the five senses,
for they lead along a ruinous course.
Give up desires and scatter them.
Attain to the Truth of wisdom:
that is the Way to reach the Lord.

Tiru-Mandiram

Instruction in Happiness

Lord Krishna said:

O Kirīti, I will set out before thy vision that happiness which is experienced when the individual soul meets the Self.

A divine medicine is taken in a small dose at stated times, and through the process of alchemy tin is transmuted into silver.

Water is poured on salt several times to make salt water.

So even the least measure of such happiness experienced by the self through training must wipe out sorrow.

This bliss of the Self is threefold in its nature, and I will describe these aspects in turn.

The happiness which is like poison at first and like nectar at the end, which springs from a clear understanding of the Self, is said to be of the nature of "goodness" (sattva). [Bhagavad-Gītā 18.37]

The roots of a sandalwood tree are dangerous owing to the presence of snakes, and there are demons at the mouth of a hole where treasures are hidden.

Laborious sacrifices must be made before reaching the pleasures of heaven; the age of childhood is beset with difficulties.

When lighting a lamp one has to endure its smoke, and when one takes medicine it may be unpleasant for the tongue.

So it is, O Pāndava, with this happiness which is obtained through the difficult exercise of control of mind and senses.

This kind of happiness is attained only after real initial difficulty; but from the churning of the ocean of milk there comes the reward of nectar.

When firm resolution, like that of the god Shiva, has swallowed the poison of dispassion, then will follow the feast of the nectar of knowledge.

Unripe grapes may sting the tongue like burning coals, but when ripe they are full of sweetness.

So when by the light of the Self dispassion is perfected, and with it ignorance in every form is destroyed,

then the intellect becomes merged in the Self as the water of the Ganges flows into the ocean, and the great store of the bliss of union is opened.

Therefore the happiness which is rooted in dispassion and leads to the experience of union is said to have the quality of goodness.

> *The happiness which arises from the contact of the senses and their objects, and which is like nectar at first but like poison at the end, is recorded to be "passionate" (rajas).*　　*[Bhagavad-Gītā 18.38]*

When the senses and sense objects are united, O conqueror of wealth, this kind of happiness overflows its banks.

When a ruler visits a town a festival is held, and money is borrowed for the celebration of a marriage.

Sugar and plantains taste equally sweet to the tongue of a sick man, and the poisonous bacnaga plant is pleasing to look at.

All such happiness comes to an end and even life may be destroyed and all accumulated merit is wasted.

All the pleasures which have been enjoyed vanish like a dream, leaving a man struck down by disaster.

Thus happiness of this kind brings about disaster in this world and turns to poison in the next.

O Pārtha, such is this happiness which is full of passion; therefore thou shouldst avoid any contact with it.

> *That happiness which deludes the soul both at the*
> *beginning and at the end, and which arises from*
> *sleep, sloth and negligence, is declared to be of the*
> *nature of "darkness" (tamas). [Bhagavad-Gītā 18.39]*

The happiness which arises from indulgence in drink, from eating undesirable food, and in the company of loose women,

from assault and robbery of others and from the praise of bards,

that is fed by sloth and enjoyed in undue sleep and which leaves a man always confused about the way he should live,

such happiness, O Pārtha, is truly of the nature of darkness. I will not say much about it, for it can hardly be experienced as happiness.

Jnāneshvarī

The Value of Contentment

Sage Nārada said:

For a person who is contented, everything is always and everywhere auspicious, just as a person wearing shoes is safe from thorns and pebbles.

O King, how can a contented person subsist on water alone? Because of the wretchedness of the genitals and the tongue, a person keeps house.

Brilliance, knowledge, asceticism, and fame fade for that brahmin who is discontented, and also his wisdom vanishes because of the fickleness of his senses.

A person can reach the end of his needs by eating and drinking or the end of his anger by seeing justice done, but not the end of his greed, even after he has conquered and enjoyed the whole world.

O King, many pundits of great learning and capable of removing doubt in others, some of whom even preside over assemblies, fall low because of their dissatisfaction.

One should conquer desire through resolution; anger through abandoning desire; greed by considering the worthlessness of material goods; fear through recollecting the Truth;

delusion and grief through deliberation; pride through service to the great ones; the obstacles to Yoga through the practice of silence; harmfulness by not favoring such desires;

suffering caused by other beings through compassion; suffering caused by destiny through ecstasy and renunciation; self-caused suffering by the potency of Yoga; sleep by cultivating the quality of lucidity.

One should conquer the qualities of passion and dullness through lucidity; and lucidity through equanimity. All this a person can do through devotion to the teacher.

Bhāgavata-Purāna

The Conquest of Desire

Desires are threefold: objective, subjective, and of the form of subconscious impressions. The tasting of sweetmeats, for instance, is objective; hoping for sweetmeats, for instance, is subjective; and desires that occur spontaneously, such as touching grass when passing over a footpath, are considered to be of the form of subconscious impressions. When one is concentrated, one abandons all desires, because one's mind is entirely devoid of movement. Such a one has contentment, as is seen in the cheerfulness of his countenance. Such contentment is to be found not in desires but only in the Self, when all desires have been abandoned and when the mind is close to the reality of the Self in the form of supreme bliss. In this state, the bliss of the Self is not experienced as one of the movements of the mind, as in conscious ecstasy *(samprajñāta-samādhi)*. Rather, it is experienced by the self-illumining Self itself, which is of the form of Consciousness. Contentment, again, is not a movement of the mind but a subconscious imprint left by that bliss.

Jīvanmukti-Viveka

The Two Streams of the Mind

The stream of the mind flows in two directions. It flows toward the good, and it flows toward the bad. The one commencing with discernment and ending in liberation flows toward the good. The one commencing with lack of discernment and ending in worldly existence (*samsāra*) flows toward the bad. Through dispassion the flux toward the sense objects is checked, and through the practice of the vision of discernment the stream of discernment is laid bare. Thus the restriction of the whirls of the mind is dependent on both [i.e., dispassion and the practice of discernment].

Yoga-Bhāshya

The Bottleneck of the Mind

People talk about freedom; people talk about salvation. What is it that has bound you first? If you want to be free, if you want to get salvation, you ought to know what is the cause of your bondage. It is just like the monkey in the fable. A monkey is caught in India in a very queer manner. A narrow-necked basin is fixed in the ground, and in that basin are put some nuts and other eatables which the monkeys like. The monkeys come up and thrust their hands into the narrow-necked basin and fill their hands with the nuts. The fist becomes thick, and it cannot be taken out. There the monkey is caught.

We ask what it is that binds you first. You yourself have brought you under thralldom and bondage. Here is the whole wide world, a grand magnificent forest; and in this grand magnificent wood of the whole universe, there is a narrow-necked vessel found. What is that narrow-necked vessel? It is your brain. Herein are some nuts and people have got hold of these nuts, and all that is done through the agency of the brain or through the medium of this intellect is owned as one's own. "I am the mind," is what everybody says; everybody has practically identified himself with the mind; "I am the mind," "I am the intellect," and he takes a strong grip of these nuts of this narrow-necked vessel. That is what makes you a slave to anxiety, a slave to fear, a slave to temptations, a slave to all sorts of troubles. That is what binds you; that is the cause of all the suffering in this world. If you want salvation, if you want freedom, only let go the hold, free your hand. The whole forest is yours; you can jump from tree to tree and eat all the nuts. The whole world is yours; just get rid of this selfish ignorance and you are free, you are your own savior.

SWAMI RAMA TIRTHA

The Power of Thought

The mind verily is the world (*samsāra*)
One should purify it strenuously.
One assumes the form of that which is in one's mind.
This is the eternal secret.

Maitrī-Upanishad

The Mind Is the Cause of Bondage and Liberation

The mind is said to be twofold; pure and impure.
The impure has desire and volition; the pure is devoid
of desire.

The mind alone is the cause of bondage and liberation
for humans.
Attached to objects, it leads to bondage; devoid of
objects, it is deemed to lead to emancipation.

Because liberation of the mind devoid of objects is
desirable,
The seeker after liberation should always make the
mind devoid of objects.

When the mind, freed from contact with objects and
restricted in the heart,
becomes nonexistent, then that is the supreme state.

It should be checked until it meets with destruction in
the heart.
This is wisdom; this is meditation. The rest is diffuse
speculation.

Amrita-Bindu-Upanishad

The Ego

What stands in the way of course is always the vital ego with its ignorance and the pride of its ignorance and the physical consciousness with its inertia which resents and resists any call to change and its indolence which does not like to take the trouble—it finds it more comfortable to go on its own way repeating always the same old movements and, at best, expecting everything to be done for it in some way or at some time.

SRI AUROBINDO

Delete the "I"-Thought through Self-Inquiry

❀

Ramana Maharshi: How do you meditate?

Questioner: I begin with asking myself "Who am I?" and eliminate the body as not "I," the breath as not "I," the mind as not "I," but then I am unable to proceed further.

Ramana Maharshi: Well, that is all right so far as the mind goes. Your process is only mental. Actually all the scriptures mention this process only in order to guide the seeker to the Truth. The Truth cannot be directly indicated; that is why this mental process is used. You see, he who eliminates all the "not-I" cannot eliminate the "I." In order to be able to say "I am not this" or "I am That," there must be the "I" to say it. This "I" is only the ego, or the "I"-thought. After the rising up of this "I"-thought, all other thoughts arise. The "I"-thought is therefore the root thought. If the root is pulled out, all the rest is at the same time uprooted. Therefore seek the root "I"; question yourself: "Who am I?"; find out the source of the "I." Then all these problems will vanish and the pure Self alone will remain.

Questioner: But how am I to do it?

Ramana Maharshi: The "I" is always there, whether in deep sleep, in dream or in the waking state. The one who sleeps is the same as the one who is now speaking. There is always the feeling of "I." If it were not so you would have to deny your existence. But you do not. You say: "I am." Find out who is.

Questioner: I still do not understand. You say the "I" is now the false "I." How am I to eliminate this wrong "I"?

Ramana Maharshi: You need not eliminate any false "I." How can "I" eliminate itself? All that you need do is to find out its origin and stay there. Your effort can extend only so far. Then the Beyond will take care of itself. You are helpless there. NO effort can reach it.

Questioner: If "I" am always—here and now—why do I not feel so?

Ramana Maharshi: Who says that you do not? Does the real "I" or the false "I"? Ask yourself and you will find that it is the false "I." The false "I" is the obstruction which has to be removed in order that the true "I" may cease to be hidden. The feeling that "I have not realized" is the obstruction to realization. In fact, it is already realized. There is nothing more to be realized. If there were, the realization would be something new which did not yet exist, but was to come about in the future; but whatever is born will also die. If realization is not eternal it is not worth having. Therefore, what we seek is not something that must begin to exist but only what is eternal but is veiled from us by obstructions. All that we need do is to remove the obstruction. What is eternal is not recognized as such owing to ignorance. Ignorance is the obstruction. Get rid of it and all will be well. This ignorance is identical with the "I"-thought. Seek its source and it will vanish.

The Teachings of Ramana Maharshi

The Five Hindrances

❀

Ignorance, I-am-ness (*asmitā*), attachment, aversion, and the will to live are the five causes of affliction.

Ignorance is the field of the others, which can be dormant, attenuated, intercepted, or aroused.

Ignorance is seeing that which is eternal, pure, joyful, and the Self in that which is ephemeral, impure, sorrowful, and the nonself.

I-am-ness is the identification as it were of the power of vision with the power of the visioner [the Self].

Attachment is that which follows pleasure.

Aversion is that which follows pain.

The will to live, flowing along by its own momentum, is rooted thus even in knowledgeable persons.

In their subtle form, these causes of affliction are to be overcome through involution.

The mental fluctuations of these [subtle forms] are to be overcome through meditation.

The causes of affliction are the root of the karmic deposit, which may be experienced in the present or during a future birth.

So long as the root exists, there is also fruition from it: birth, life, and experience.

These result in delight or distress, depending on the karmic causes, which may be meritorious or demeritorious.

Because of the suffering inherent in change, in anguish, and in the subconscious factors, and on account of the conflict between the movements of the primary constituents of nature, to the discerning person all is but suffering.

What is to be overcome is future suffering.

Yoga-Sūtra

Mental Restlessness

Sage Vasishtha said:

Wherever one looks, there is no movement in this world without the mind. Restlessness is the quality of the mind, just as heat is the quality of fire.

Indeed, know this power of vibratory movement, which characterizes consciousness, to be the mental power and identical with the apex of the world.

Just as wind does not exist apart from vibration together with stillness, so also consciousness does not exist without vibratory movement.

That which is without motion is called the dead mind. And that is indeed asceticism, the fulfillment of the scriptures, or liberation.

Only through the absorption of the mind is peace from suffering found. By means of the thinking mind, however, only much suffering is harvested.

The demon of the mind, once roused, brings up suffering. Energetically put it to rest to experience infinite joy.

O Rāma, its restlessness is what is called ignorance. By means of discrimination destroy that which is merely subconscious tendencies and verbal designations.

By the power of renunciation, which dissolves the mind together with ignorance and the endless subconscious tendencies, one attains the supreme good.

O Rāma, that which is between existence and nonexistence and between sentience and insentience, always swinging between both extremes, is called the mind.

When lost in contemplating the insentient, the mind assumes the nature of insentience and thus becomes insentient itself by force of solid repetition.

However, by contemplating only with discernment, which is of the nature of a fragment of Consciousness, the mind, likewise by force of solid repetition, achieves union with Consciousness.

Through practice, the mind reaches whatever condition it is focused upon with manly effort, and then becomes it.

Relying on your human mind and taking refuge in the sorrowless condition, with resolute intent and without fear, become stable.

O Rāma, if the mind, which is immersed in the contemplation of existence, is not forcibly uplifted by means of the mind alone, then there is no other means.

Only the mind, O Rāghava, is capable of firmly restraining the mind; for who is capable of disciplining a king if not a king?

Yoga-Vāsishtha

Tether the Mind

The steed called mind roams space,
covering one hundred thousand miles
in the blink of an eye.
He who does not know how to tether it
is apt to be battered to death
by the inbreath and the outbreath.

LALLĀ

Be Grateful to the Mind

The mind cannot find perfect repose anywhere except in God. When you meet God, you find everything, and the mind becomes steady. Then, even if you try, it doesn't move. From this point of view, it is the restlessness of your mind that has never been satisfied by temporary stillness, which has set you on the search for truth and peace. . . . You should consider this a great service on the part of the mind. The restlessness of your mind is a great asset to you, for it has fostered your interest in meditation and has made you worthy of the grace of the Siddhas [adepts]. So you should welcome heartily the beneficent grace of the mind.

SWAMI MUKTANANDA

The Steed of the Mind

I'll put the bit and bridle
On you, O steed of my mind;
Discarding all else
I'll gallop you toward Gagan [inner space].

Self-realization is my saddle;
In the stirrup of Sahaj
I place my foot and ride,
Astride the steed of my mind.

Come, my steed, I'll take you
On a trip to heaven;
If you balk
I'll urge you on
With the whip of divine love.

KABĪR

Three Great Obstacles on the Path

There are many defects (*dosha*) in the mind that are destructive of everything. Because of them, people are constantly stewing in the terrible world of change.

The first of these defects is lack of conviction; the second, the tendency of desire; and the third, dullness. These are said to be the threefold collection of the defects.

Lack of conviction, which is twofold, consists of doubt and misconception about whether liberation is or is not true. First, doubt arises

that liberation may not be true; then there is a misconception about it. Both are the principal blocks to true intent.

One should gradually eliminate both by means of considering their opposites. This is the foremost means, and nothing else can cut them at the root.

Now, the root of lack of conviction is faulty reasoning. Give it up to achieve a properly reasoned approach.

Consideration of the opposites should aim at cutting their root. Then lack of conviction vanishes through the growth of faith.

The root tendency of desire prevents the mind from hearing the truth. A mind embroiled in the root tendency of desire cannot advance.

Indeed, in the world, a desirer is always intent on contemplating his desires, so that he cannot see what is in front of him and cannot hear what is said even within earshot.

For a person in the grip of the root tendency of desire, sacred tradition (*shruta*) is the same as that which is not sacred tradition. Therefore the root tendency of desire must be conquered by means of complete dispassion.

The tendencies, which are headed by desire and anger, are thousandfold. Desire is the root of them. When it is removed, none remain.

Therefore one should eliminate the tendency of desire by engaging in dispassion. Even hope is said to be a form of desire unless placed in Me.

According to the foremost of seers, the third defect of the mind, which takes the form of dullness, is virtually impossible to conquer by practice.

In this case, there is no other means except service to the divinity of the Self.

Tripura-Rahasya

The Fault of Indecisiveness

The woman sage Cūdālā said:

There was a fortunate man who enjoyed the truly con-
tradictory situation of both virtue and wealth, similar
to the world ocean combining water and fire.

Gifted, skillful in arms, careful in his dealings, he
achieved all his purposes but did not know the
Supreme.

To obtain the wish-fulfilling gem, he applied himself
with infinite effort, rather as the subterranean fire fi-
nally dries out the ocean.

Because of his great effort and firm resolution over
time, the wish-fulfilling gem appeared to him. What
cannot be accomplished by oneself if one but tries?

When effort is combined with intelligence, a person
who is energetic, even if poverty-stricken, will attain
his potential unhindered.

He saw the gem lying close before him within the reach of his hands, just as the rising moon is for a sage on a mountain peak.

The brilliant gem was there, but he became uncertain, like a poor person who one good day found himself to be the king.

For hours he thought about the miraculous stone, ignoring that he had actually obtained the elusive stone that had involved him in long tribulation.

"Is this the stone or is it not the stone? If it is, then how can it possibly be it? Should I touch it or should I not touch it? Will it vanish if I touch it?

"Surely one cannot obtain that most excellent gem in such a short time. According to tradition, one can obtain it only after a whole life of striving.

"I see this shining gem only because I am a miser, just as one sees waving lights with closed eyes and just as one sees a double moon because of faulty vision.

"How could good fortune come my way so easily, that I should now obtain that most excellent gem, which bestows all powers?

"Few indeed must be those fortunate ones for whom fortune approaches after such a short time.

"I am a quite wretched man of few austerities. How can these powers come to me by sheer good fortune?"

Thus that ignoramus was gripped by doubt and speculation. Deluded by his stupidity, he made no effort to grasp the gem.

While he was in this confused state, the gem disappeared and the powers abandoned him, just as one avoids a scoffer or an arrow shot from a bowstring.

Yoga-Vāsishtha

The Metaphor of the Chariot

Know the Self as the master of the chariot and the body as the chariot. Know wisdom (*buddhi*) as the charioteer and the mind as the reins.

The senses, they say, are the horses; the sense objects are their paths. The Self associated with the senses and the mind the sages call the "enjoyer."

He who is ignorant and always has an undisciplined mind, his senses are uncontrolled as bad-tempered horses are for a charioteer.

But he who understands and always has a disciplined mind, his senses are controlled as well-behaved horses are for a charioteer.

He who lacks understanding and is always inattentive and impure does not attain the highest state but remains in cyclic existence (*samsāra*).

But he who understands and is always attentive and pure attains that state whereupon he is not reborn.

Katha-Upanishad

The Nature of Knowledge

Lord Krishna said:

Lack of pride, unpretentiousness, nonharming,
patience, uprightness, reverence for one's teacher,
purity, steadiness, self-restraint,

dispassion toward the sense objects, lack of ego sense,
insight into the flaws of birth, death, old age, illness,
and suffering,

nonattachment, absence of clinging to offspring, wife,
home, and the like, and a constant same-mindedness
(*sama-cittatva*) in desirable and undesirable circum-
stances,

as well as unswerving devotion to Me by means of the
Yoga of non-otherness, resorting to a solitary place,
dislike for social contact,

constancy in the knowledge concerning the Self, and
insight into the purpose of knowledge of reality—this
is called knowledge. Ignorance is that which is other
than this.

Bhagavad-Gītā

Self-Knowledge

Questioner: How can one know the "I"?

Ramana Maharshi: The "I" is always there. There is no knowing it. It is not a new knowledge acquired. What is new and not here and now will be evanescent only. The "I" is always there. There is obstruction to its knowledge and it is called ignorance. Remove the ignorance and knowledge shines forth. In fact, this ignorance or knowledge does not relate to the Self. They are only overgrowth to be cleared away. That is why the Self is said to be beyond knowledge and ignorance. It remains as it naturally is—that is all.

Talks with Sri Ramana Maharshi

Yoga and Wisdom

❀

Wisdom is generated by Yoga; Yoga is produced by wisdom.

That yogi who is ever intent on Yoga and wisdom does not perish. He should behold Shiva abiding in all change but see no change in Shiva.

Thinking of nothing else, he should contemplate by means of Yoga that which is revealed by Yoga. He who does not possess Yoga and wisdom is unable to reach the state of liberation.

Therefore the yogi should restrain the mind and the vital energies (*prāna*) by means of the Yoga of practice and should sever them as with a keen-edged blade.

Trishikhi-Brāhmana-Upanishad

The Ultimate Futility of Intellectual Learning

Lord Shiva said:

O Beloved! Creatures have fallen into the deep well of the six schools of philosophy, but controlled by the fetters of creatures, they do not know the supreme Reality.

Struggling in the terrible ocean of the Vedic scriptures, they are seized by monsters in the waves of time and remain there through faulty reasoning.

He who knows the Vedas, Āgamas, and Purānas but does not know the supreme Reality, for such an imitator everything is meaningless crow's cawing.

Full of ideas like "This is knowledge" and "This is to be known," they study day and night, O Goddess, while facing away from the supreme Truth.

Afflicted by concerns over syntax, arguments, prosody, and composition, and adorned with the ornaments of poetry, these fools have their senses confused.

The supreme Truth is one thing and how people are afflicted is another. The true state described in the texts is one thing and the explanations they give are another.

They talk about the transmental state but do not experience it for themselves. Some, who are bereft of instruction, even succumb to the ego (*ahamkāra*).

They study the Vedic texts and argue with each other, but they do not know the supreme Truth, just as a serpent is unaware of the venom it generates.

The head carries the flowers but the nose smells their scent. They study the Vedic texts, but knowledge of their Reality is difficult to attain.

Ignorant about the Truth within himself, the fool becomes lost in the texts just as a foolish shepherd looks for a billy goat in a well when it has already returned to the pen.

Verbal knowledge is not sufficient for removing the delusion of the world, just as darkness cannot be dispelled by mere talk of a lamp.

The study of someone lacking in wisdom is like the mirror image of a blind person. O Goddess, only for those endowed with wisdom are the scriptures a source of true knowledge.

Kula-Arnava-Tantra

Book Knowledge versus Self-Knowledge

The sage Durvāsas came with a bundle of textbooks to pay homage to Mahādeva. When in the assembly of that god, Sage Nārada compared him to an ass carrying a load. Angrily he threw his books into the salty ocean, whereupon Mahādeva imparted to him knowledge of the Self (*ātma-vidyā*). Self-knowledge is not attained by someone who is not introspective and lacks the teacher's grace. Thus scripture [*Katha-Upanishad* 1.2.22] states: "This Self is not attained by discussion, intelligence, or learning."

Jīvanmukti-Viveka

The Need for Discipline

It is necessary to practice some spiritual discipline. The guru no doubt does everything for the disciple; but at the end he makes the disciple work a little himself. When cutting down a big tree, a man cuts almost through the trunk; then he stands aside for a moment, and the tree falls down with a crash.

The farmer brings water to his field through a canal from the river. He stands aside when only a little digging remains to be done to connect the field with the water. Then the earth becomes soaked and falls of itself, and the water of the river pours into the canal in torrents.

A man is able to see God as soon as he gets rid of ego and other limitations. He sees God as soon as he is free from such feelings as "I am a scholar," "I am the son of such and such a person," "I am wealthy," "I am honorable," and so forth.

"God alone is real and all else unreal; the world is illusory"—that is discrimination. One cannot assimilate spiritual instruction without discrimination.

Through the practice of spiritual discipline one attains perfection, by the grace of God. But one must also labor a little. Then one sees God and enjoys bliss. If a man hears that a jar filled with gold is buried at a certain place, he rushes there and begins to dig. He sweats as he goes on digging. After much digging he feels the spade strike something. Then he throws away the spade and looks for the jar. At the sight of the jar he dances for joy. Then he takes up the jar and pours out the gold coins. He takes them into his hand, counts them, and feels the ecstasy of joy. Vision—touch—enjoyment. Isn't it so?

SRI RAMAKRISHNA

Making Time for the Divine

I find people complaining that they do not find time for worship or meditation. But I feel, and everybody knows well, that they always get sufficient time for their illness, worries and physical needs. The reason is that all these things are of greater importance to them than the Divine duties. As a matter of fact a man can keep himself busy with divine thoughts every moment without offering any hindrance to his worldly activities. If one practices it so as to form his habit it becomes so easy and natural with him that he would not like to part with it even for a moment. I give you all a very helpful hint. Before taking up a certain work, think of Him for a while in the sense that He himself is doing it. It is the simplest method and I should like you all to follow it in right earnest.

RAM CHANDRA

Practice Makes Perfect

The Blessed Goddess said:

Whenever one does anything, one has no success whatsoever without practice (*abhyāsa*).

The sages know this to be practice: being dedicated to one thing, reflecting upon it, talking about it with one another, and understanding it.

The great souls, having renounced the world, accomplish the reduction of fondness for pleasure and, while here on Earth, attain the highest state.

The mind of those practitioners (*abhyāsin*) who delight in the flavor of renunciation even in regard to the greatest beauty is vibrant with bliss.

Upon succeeding in the total negation of knower and knowable objects, those who are guided by reason and the textbooks are established as practitioners of the Absolute (*brahman*).

The practice of understanding is explained to consist in the notions that nothing was ever created, visible objects have never existed, and I am this world.

The practice of the Absolute is explained to consist in the attenuation of attachment, aversion, and so on by means of understanding the nonexistence of visible objects upon the strong dawning of delight.

The attenuation of aversion and so on unaccompanied by understanding the nonexistence of visible objects is called asceticism. Therefore there is no wisdom, only suffering.

Understanding the nonexistence of visible objects is indeed called wisdom worthy to be known. By such practice comes extinction (*nirvāna*). This indeed is practice, the great dawn.

Yoga-Vāsishtha

Daily Discipline

❧

After practicing Yoga for one *ghatikā* (twenty-four minutes) or one *muhūrta* (forty-eight minutes) according to one's capacity, then spending one *muhūrta* listening to teachings or attending to the teacher, taking care of bodily needs for the next *muhūrta,* and thereafter studying Yoga teachings for another *muhūrta,* one should practice again Yoga for one *muhūrta.* Thus giving prominence to Yoga in all one's daily activities, one should combine them with it and carry them out promptly. At bedtime, one should count the *muhūrtas* spent in Yoga during the day. Then one should increase the time devoted to Yoga during the next day or the next fortnight or the next month. When the time devoted to Yoga is thus increased even by an instant for every *muhūrta,* at the end of a year the time devoted to Yoga will have increased. That exclusive dedication to Yoga leaves no room for other activities need not be doubted. Fitness in Yoga comes to those who are completely free from all other activities. Accordingly, the renunciation of the knower is preferred. Hence one who is exclusively devoted to this becomes, stage by stage, one who has ascended Yoga (*yoga-ārūdha*).

Jīvanmukti-Viveka

Asceticism Is Everything

The threefold universe is pervaded by asceticism (*tapas*), radiant in all beings. Through asceticism, the sun and the moon shine in the heavens.

The splendor of asceticism is wisdom. Asceticism is what is talked about in the world. Whatever action removes passion (*rajas*) and lethargy (*tamas*) is essentially asceticism.

Chastity and nonharming are said to be asceticism of the body. Restraint of thought and speech are similarly said to be asceticism of the mind.

Mahābhārata

Success in Yoga

Success, for certain, comes to a person who has faith in the Self. There is no success for others. Therefore one should make every effort to practice.

Those who are fond of learning, lack confidence, fail to pay homage to the teacher, and have numerous concerns,

as well as who are fond of deceitful talk and harsh language and fail to please the teacher, can never be successful.

Confidence that their efforts will bear fruit is the first sign of success. The second is being filled with faith; the third reverence for the teacher;

the fourth is the state of equanimity; the fifth is control of the five senses; and the sixth is moderate diet. There is no seventh.

Shiva-Samhitā

The True Guru

Let the disciple have confidence in himself
And speak with understanding;
What he says will come to pass—if first we cry to God.

Do as the True Guru bids you, if you are a wise disciple.
Whither he has brought you, there remain steadfast:
Why ask foolish questions?

The Guru speaks first with the mind,
Then with a glance of the eye;
If the disciple fails to understand,
He instructs him at last by word of mouth.

He who understands the spoken word is a common man;
He who interprets a gesture is an initiate;
He who reads the thoughts of the mind,
Unsearchable, unfathomable, is a divinity.

My tongue is forever speaking:
Your ears are continually hearing.
But what can the poor True Guru do
If his pupil is an ignorant fool?

Dādū

Characteristics of a Superior Teacher

❀

Lord Shiva said:

He who bestows the understanding that "I am the knower of the essence of the teachings," "I am the seed," and who is not cut off from the Divine and ever content in the heart—he is said to be a guru.

He who is indifferent to the stages of life and social classes and who, always abiding in the Self alone, has the Light for his stage of life and social class—that yogi, O Beloved, is spoken of as a guru.

He whose gaze is firm even without objects, whose mind is stable without support, and whose life force (*vāyu*) is stable without effort—he, O Beloved, is a guru.

He who knows the truth born of awareness and arising from supreme bliss—he, O Noble Lady, is a guru.

He who knows, in actuality, the state of oneness between the microcosm and the macrocosm, as well as head, bones, and the number of hairs—he and none other, O Beloved, is a guru.

Hatred, doubt, fear, shame, and, fifthly, disgust, as well as family, conduct, and caste are described as the eight bonds.

He who is bound by these bonds is to be known as a "beast" (*pashu*); he who is released from these bonds is the Great Lord. Hence he who removes these bonds is deemed a supreme guru.

Gurus are as numerous as lamps in every house. But, O Goddess, difficult to find is a guru who lights up everything like the Sun.

Gurus who are proficient in the Vedas, textbooks, and so on, are numerous. But, O Goddess, difficult to find is a guru who is proficient in the supreme Truth.

Gurus who know petty mantras and herbal concoctions are numerous. But difficult to find here on earth is one who knows the mantras described in the Nigamas, Āgamas, and textbooks.

Gurus who rob their disciples of their wealth are numerous. But, O Goddess, difficult to find is a guru who removes his disciples' suffering.

Numerous here on Earth are those who are intent on social class, stage of life, and family. But he who is devoid of all concerns is a guru difficult to find.

An intelligent man should choose a guru by whose contact supreme bliss is produced, and only such a guru and none other.

One is liberated by him whose mere sight keeps the mind active until realization (*anubhava*). There is no doubt about this.

The triple realm of movable and immovable things is completely devoured by doubt. But he who has devoured that doubt is known as a guru difficult to find.

Just as butter melts when it is close to fire, so sin dissolves when brought close to the eternal teacher.

Just as a lighted fire burns up wood, whether dry or damp, so the guru's glance burns up a disciple's sin in an instant.

Just as a cotton ball flung high by a great wind is scattered in the ten directions, so the disciple's heap of sins disappears through the guru's compassion.

Just as darkness is dispelled by the mere appearance of light, so ignorance is destroyed by the mere appearance of the true guru.

The knower of Truth, even though he may be lacking all identifying characteristics, is known as a guru. Therefore the knower of Truth alone is liberated and a liberator.

The knower of Truth, O Great Goddess, illumines even a beast. But how can one grasp the knowledge of the Truth of the inner Self when one lacks the Truth?

Those who are instructed by a knower of Truth, they become knowers of Truth. There is no doubt about this. However, those who are instructed by beasts, O Goddess, are known to become beasts themselves.

Kula-Arnava-Tantra

Three Kinds of Preceptor

The impeller, the awakener, and the bestower of liberation who is remembered as the Supreme:

These are to be known as the three kinds of preceptor on this earth. The impeller shows the path. The awakener points to the Abode. The bestower of liberation *is* the supreme Truth, knowing which one enjoys immortality.

Brahma-Vidyā-Upanishad

Characteristics of a Disciple

Lord Shiva said:

O Noble Mistress! A good disciple should be endowed
with auspicious characteristics, qualified for the practice
(*sādhana*) of ecstasy, possessed of virtuous behavior,

clean in body and garment, wise, just, pure-minded,
steady in his vows, of good conduct, possessed of faith
and devotion,

skillful, eating sparsely, thinking deeply, serving hon-
estly, acting maturely, heroic, free from mental poverty,

very skillful in all actions, pure, helpful to all, grateful,
fearful of sin, frequenting virtuous ascetics (*sādhu*),
thoughtful,

honoring tradition (*āstika*), practicing generosity,
dedicated to the welfare of all beings, equipped with
trust and discipline, not deceitful about wealth, body,
and so on,

accomplishing the impossible, brave, endowed with strength and energy, well disposed, oriented toward action, attentive, discerning,

speaking moderately and with a smile what is good and true, free from blemishes, capable of grasping what is said to him, dexterous, of broad understanding,

indifferent to praise but open, O Beloved, to criticism from others, with his senses mastered, well contented, intelligent, chaste,

as well as free from worry, sickness, instability, suffering, delusion, and doubt.

Kula-Arnava-Tantra

Four Types of Yoga Practitioners

He who is unenthusiastic, quite foolish, sickly, slandering the teacher, greedy, of wicked mind, overeating, consorting with women,

fickle, timid, diseased, dependent on others, very rude, and ill-mannered should be known as a weak practitioner (*sādhaka*).

Success will come to him after twelve years of extreme effort. The teacher should, to be sure, regard him as fit for *mantra-yoga*.

He who is even-minded, endowed with patience, intent on merit, soft-spoken, neutral, and without a doubt equal in all activities—

to him (who is a middling practitioner) the teacher, understanding this, skillfully imparts *laya-yoga*.

He who has a stable mind, applying himself to *laya-yoga*, is self-reliant, energetic, high-minded, endowed with compassion, forebearing, truthful, courageous, with faith in *laya-yoga*, worshiping the teacher's lotus feet, and fond of Yoga practice should be known as a special practitioner.

To him the wise teacher imparts *hatha-yoga* entirely. Success will come to him after six years of Yoga practice.

He who is endowed with great energy, is enthusiastic, charming, heroic, learned, disposed to practice, free from delusion, unperturbed,

full of youthful vigor, eating moderately, with senses controlled, fearless, pure, efficient, giving, a refuge for everyone,

competent, steady, wise, knowing his own mind, patient, well behaved, of virtuous conduct, doing noble deeds secretly, polite,

peaceful, endowed with confidence, worshiping the teacher and the deities, shunning social gatherings, and free from major illnesses—

for such a very special practitioner of all Yogas, who keeps his vows, success comes within three years for certain.

Shiva-Samhitā

The Need for Initiation

Lord Shiva said:

Initiation is the root of all victory. Initiation is the root of supreme asceticism. Initiation bestowed by a teacher accomplishes all actions.

O Beloved, the efforts of those who practice recitation (*japa*), worship (*pūja*), and other rituals but are uninitiated remain fruitless, like seed that has fallen on rock.

O Goddess! He who is bereft of initiation can have no success and no fortunate destiny. Therefore one should endeavor to seek initiation from a teacher.

Mantra-Yoga-Samhitā

Kinds of Initiation

Lord Shiva said:

According to Shiva's instruction, there can be no liberation without initiation, and there can be no initiation without a preceptor and preceptorial lineage.

Therefore, after acquiring the teachings by means of one's tradition and the like, one should find one's inner teacher; otherwise the mantras cannot be fruitful.

If, out of delusion, fear, or a desire for wealth, one initiates someone who is unfit, one invites the curse of deities, and one's work will be fruitless.

O Goddess, great Mistress, divine initiation is said to be threefold: by touch, by sight, and by thought; these are without effort and rituals.

O Beloved, instruction and initiation by touch are said to be like fledglings that are gradually made to grow by the warmth of a mother bird's wings.

O supreme Goddess, instruction and initiation by sight
are like a fish fostering its young by sight alone.

Penetrating instruction and initiation by thought are
like a tortoise caring for its offspring by mere contemplation.

The disciple is favored by receiving the descent of the
power (*shakti-pāta*). Where the power does not
descend, there is no success.

O Goddess, initiation bestowing liberation is proclaimed to be sevenfold: through ritual, the alphabet,
emanation, touch, speech, sight, and thought.

Kula-Arnava-Tantra

Good Company

I walk with those who go after God.
I live with those who sing His praise.
The Lord blesses those who seek Him.
With them I consort. Their feet I seek.

Tiru-Mandiram

Association with Holy Folk

Sage Vasishtha said:

O greatly wise Rāma, association with holy folk everywhere efficiently assists people wanting to cross over the world of change.

Association with holy folk produces the bright flower of discernment (*viveka*). Those great souls who cherish it have good fortune.

In the company of wise folk, misfortune appears as fortune, empty space as if it were populated, and death as a festival.

In this world, association with holy folk conquers the wind of delusion and the ice creeping into the lotus of the heart.

Know association with holy folk to be the best furtherance of understanding. It fells the tree of ignorance and removes the afflictions.

Association with holy folk produces the lamp of supreme discernment shining forth beautifully like a cluster of blooms after rain.

The influence of assocation with holy folk teaches us the most excellent conduct, which is safe, unobstructed, and always full.

Even though people may experience terrible conditions or find themselves in a helpless situation, they should definitely not stop seeking association with holy folk.

In this world, association with holy folk is a light upon the right path. It dispels the darkness of the heart by means of the luminosity of the sun of wisdom.

Yoga-Vāsishtha

The Path to Liberation

Sage Bhīshma said:

The path to the Western Ocean does not lead to the Eastern. Verily, the path of liberation is singular. Listen to my detailed account.

Through patience, the sage should lop off anger; through abandoning volition (*samkalpa*), he should conquer desire. Through cultivating the quality of lucidity (*sattva*), he should strive to overcome sleep.

Through attentiveness, he should protect against fear; through behaving as the knower of the field (*kshetra-jna*), he should control the breath. He should dispel self-will (*icchā*), aversion, and desire.

Through steady practice, he should dispel error, delusion, and confusion. Through the practice of wisdom, the knower of truth should conquer sleep and hallucination (*pratibhā*).

Through easily digestible moderate food, he should conquer infirmities and illnesses. Through contentment, he should overcome greed and delusion. Through the vision of reality, he should overcome the objective world.

Through compassion (*anukrosha*), he should conquer vice. Through indifference, he should conquer virtue. Through restraint, he should conquer hope. Through abstention from attachment, he should conquer wealth.

The knowledgeable one should conquer attachment by considering impermanence, hunger by means of Yoga, his own pride by means of compassion (*karunā*), and craving by being contented.

He should conquer laziness by means of exertion. He should conquer doubt through certainty and talkativeness through silence. He should conquer fear by valor.

He should control speech and mind by means of understanding (*buddhi*), and he should control that understanding by means of the eye of wisdom. The great person should control that wisdom, and he should control that which is Self's peace.

This is to be known by means of tranquillity and pure works, thus overcoming the five impediments (*dosha*) of Yoga, which the sages know well.

Abandoning desire, anger, greed, fear, and sleep as the fifth, one should pursue the right course through the practice (*sādhana*) of Yoga.

Meditation, study (*adhyayana*), generosity, truthfulness, modesty, rectitude, patience, dietary purity, purity of the senses, and restraint—

these enhance one's energy (*tejas*) and dispel one's sins. Also, they fulfill one's wishes and increase one's knowledge.

Mahābhārata

Intending Liberation

Thus you will find that intentness on great liberation is the means to it. When this intentness is full no other means is necessary.

But when intentness is weak what is the use of a thousand means? Therefore the principal means to liberation is intentness alone.

Tripura-Rahasya

Think of Yourself as Immortal

Death is a joke to me. Man stands on the glory of his own soul, the infinite, the eternal, the deathless—that soul which no instruments can pierce, which no air can dry, no fire burn, no water melt, the infinite, the birthless, the deathless, without beginning and without end, before whose magnitude the suns and moons and all their systems appear like drops in the ocean, before whose glory space melts away into nothingness and time vanishes into non-existence. This glorious soul we must believe in. Out of that will come power. Whatever you think, that you will be. If you think yourselves weak, weak you will be. If you think yourselves strong, strong you will be; if you think yourselves impure, impure you will be; if you think yourselves pure, pure you will be. This teaches us not to think of ourselves as weak, but as strong, omnipotent, omniscient. No matter that I have not expressed it yet, it is in me. All knowledge is in me, all power, all purity, and all freedom.

SWAMI VIVEKANANDA

The Caged Nightingale

There was a cage formed of mirrors,
With a fresh rose hanging in the middle.
The flower was one, but each reflection
Was a separate object of love
To the nightingale caged within.
Every time the nightingale flew towards a flower,
It received a rap.
What it thought was a flower
Was only a reflection.
When it flew towards it,
It knocked its head against the glass.
When it looked to the right,
There was the rose.
When it ran to the left,
It suffered the same fate.
When it flew forward
It stubbed its beak.
And when it fell
It received another wound.
But once it turned back
And lifted up its eyes,

There was the real rose smiling.
Feeling startled, it thought
"Let there be no more deception.
Is this a real rose
Or a rose only in name?"
It flew up at once to the rose.
Now there was joy, no cage, no mirrors.
It was free.
O Man, this is your condition
Encompassed by the cage of the world.
He in search of whom
You are wandering from door to door
Is shining peacefully within your heart.

SWAMI RAMA TIRTHA

The Inner Treasure

I have found something,
Something rare have I found;
Its value none can assess.

It has no color, it is one,
Indivisible and everlasting—
Untouched by the waves of change,
It fills each and every vessel.

It has no weight, it has no price;
Beyond the bounds of measurement,
It cannot be counted,
And through erudition
It cannot be known.
It is neither heavy nor light,
No touchstone can assay its worth.

I dwell in it, it dwells in me,
We are one, like water
Mixed with water.
He who knows it,

Will never die;
He who knows it not,
Dies again and again.

Kabīr, the Lord's slave, has discovered
An ocean filled with the nectar of love;
But I find no one disposed to taste it.
When men do not believe my words,
Words from my own experience,
What else can I say to convince them?

KABĪR

Yoga and the Divine Life

To enter the spiritual life means to take a plunge into the Divine, as you would jump into the sea. And that is not the end but the very beginning; for after you have taken the plunge, you must learn to live in the Divine. That is the plunge you have to take, and unless you do it, you may do Yoga for years and yet know nothing of a true spiritual living.

Yoga means union with the Divine, and the union is effected through offering—it is founded on the offering of yourself to the Divine. When the resolution has been taken, when you have decided that the whole of your life shall be given to the Divine, you have still at every moment to remember it and carry it out in all the details of your existence.

In the beginning of the Yoga you are apt to forget the divine very often. But by constant aspiration you increase your remembrance and you diminish the forgetfulness. But this should not be done as a severe discipline or a duty; it must be a movement of love and joy.

SRI AUROBINDO

The Foundation of Faith

Faith is clarity of the mind; like a good mother, it protects the yogi. He who thus has faith and is intent on discernment acquires energy. He who is endowed with energy gains mindfulness. And when mindfulness is present, the mind becomes undistracted and concentrated. He whose mind is concentrated attains discerning wisdom by which he perceives reality as it really is.

Yoga-Bhāshya

The Supreme Value of Faith

Arjuna said:

What, O Krishna, is the stand of those who, discarding scriptural rules, sacrifice with faith? *Sattva*, *rajas*, or *tamas*?

The Blessed One said:

The faith of embodied beings (*dehin*), which arises from their inner being, is threefold: *sattva*-natured, *rajas*-natured, and *tamas*-natured. Hear about them.

O Son of Bharata, everyone's faith is in accordance with his essence. The human being (*purusha*) is of the form of faith. Whatever his faith is, that indeed is he.

The *sattva*-natured worship the deities and the *rajas*-natured the demigods and spirits. The others, the *tamas*-natured people, worship the departed and hosts of elementals.

Bhagavad-Gītā

The Eight Limbs of Yoga

❀

Through application of the limbs of Yoga and with
the dwindling of impurity there is radiance of wis-
dom up to the vision of discernment.

The limbs of Yoga are the eight to be described. From
their application results the dwindling or removal of the
fivefold misconception, which is of the form of impurity. Upon the dwindling of this comes the manifestation
of correct knowledge (*samyag-jnāna*). According to the
means employed, the impurity is brought to a state of
attenuation. And as it dwindles, so the light of knowledge increases in keeping with the process of dwindling.
Now this increase comes to a point of perfection in the
vision of discernment (*viveka-khyāti*). It reaches up to
the perception distinguishing between the essential
form of the primary qualities (*guna*) and the Self
(*purusha*). Application of the limbs of Yoga is the cause
of the separation (*viyoga*) from impurity, just as an axe
fells a tree to be cut down. Now these are the cause of
attaining the vision of discernment, just as virtue is the
cause of happiness.

Moral discipline, self-restraint, posture, breath con-trol, sensory inhibition, concentration, meditation, and ecstasy are the eight limbs.

Application to these must happen in succession.

Yoga-Sūtra with *Yoga-Bhāshya*

The Eightfold Path

Dispassion relative to the bodily organs is called
  restraint (*yama*) by the wise.

Constant adherence to the ultimate Truth is known as
  discipline (*niyama*).
The state of indifference to all things is the foremost
  posture (*āsana*).

The faith that the whole world is false is breath control
  (*prāna-samyama*).
The mind's inward-facing condition, O best one, is
  sense withdrawal (*pratyāhāra*).

The mind's stable condition is known as holding, or
  concentration (*dhāranā*).
The thought "I am pure Awareness" is called meditation (*dhyāna*).

The complete forgetting of meditation is described as
  ecstasy (*samādhi*).

Trishiki-Brāhmana-Upanishad

The Middle Path

Unless you are established in the middle path, you have
no wisdom.
To those who are in the middle path, hell does not open
its gates.
Those who are established in the middle path are
divinities.
In the noble fellowship of the just, I too walked on
their path.

Some became saintly because they were established in
the middle path.
Some became divinities because they stood in justice.
Some attained to the state of Shiva because they stood
in justice.
And so in the noble fellowship of the just, I too stood
unfalteringly.

Tiru-Mandiram

The Path Is Difficult

Sage Bhīshma said:

This path of the knowledgeable brahmins is difficult to tread. No one, O Bhāratarshabha, can walk it easily.

It is like a terrifying, difficult-to-traverse forest that has many snakes, creeping creatures, and pits, as well as numerous thorns but no water.

Or it is like a forest without edibles, or with its soil burned after a forest fire, or like a path abounding in robbers which only young men can traverse safely.

Mahābhārata

Spontaneity

Blind one,
How can you stumble
On a straight,
Spontaneous path?
Be spontaneous
In your own self,
And find the way
That is born in you . . .

JĀDUBINDU

Freedom in Action

Lord Krishna said:

Not by abstaining from actions does a man enjoy action-transcendence (*naishkarmya*), nor does he approach perfection by mere renunciation.

For not even for a moment can anyone remain without performing actions. Everyone is unwittingly made to act by the primary qualities (*guna*) born of nature.

He who restrains his organs of action but goes on remembering in his mind the objects of the senses is called a self-bewildered hypocrite.

But more excellent is he, O Arjuna, who, controlling with his mind the senses, embarks unattached on the Yoga of Action (*karma-yoga*) with his organs of action.

You must do the allotted actions, for action is superior to inaction; not even your body's processes can be accomplished by inaction.

This world is bound by action, unless one's actions are intended as a sacrifice. With that purpose, O Kaunteya, engage in action devoid of attachment.

Therefore always perform, unattached, the work to be done, for the man who performs actions without attachment attains the Supreme.

Indeed, by action did King Janaka and others attain complete perfection. Even considering only the world's welfare, you ought to act.

Whatever the best person does, that verily other people do as well. The world follows the standard such a one sets for himself.

For Me, O Pārtha, there is nothing to be done in the three worlds, nothing ungained to be gained—yet I engage in action constantly.

For if I were not untiringly to abide in action, people would, O Pārtha, follow everywhere My "track."

If I were not to perform actions, these worlds would perish, and I would be the author of chaos destroying [all] these creatures.

Always performing all actions and taking refuge in Me, he attains through My grace the eternal, immutable State.

Renouncing in thought all actions to Me, intent on Me, resorting to *buddhi-yoga*, be constantly Me-minded!

Being Me-minded, you will transcend all obstacles by My grace. But if out of ego sense (*ahamkāra*) you will not listen, then you will perish.

Bhagavad-Gītā

Commune with Nature

Smile with the flower and the green grass. Play with the butterflies, birds, and deer. Shake hands with the shrubs, ferns, and twigs of trees. Talk to the rainbow, wind, stars, and the sun. Converse with the running brooks and the waves of the sea. Speak with the walking-stick. Develop friendship with all your neighbours, dogs, cats, cows, human beings, trees, flowers, etc. Then you will have a wide, perfect, rich, full life. You will realise oneness or unity of life. This can be hardly described in words. You will have to feel this yourself.

SWAMI SIVANANDA

Channeling Emotions

Emotions in themselves are not bad, but when running wild they can be extremely damaging. Even love, when not shared, not given freely and generously, becomes self-love which turns destructively back on the individual. When emotions are directed, they are a source of strength for great achievements. Through the power of emotions men and women have overcome their limitations and attained a higher purpose in life. Emotions channeled through a Mantra towards the Divine can take you close to God.

Swami Sivananda Radha

Base Emotions

Neither heaven nor liberation can be attained by a man of base emotion even if he were to immolate himself in the sacred fire. The only result would be that his body would burn up completely.

We assert that a person of base desire and feeling never becomes pure, even if he were to do ablutions throughout his life with all the waters of the Ganges and a mountain of sand.

If a person of defiled emotion were to immolate himself by entering a huge blazing fire kindled by sprinkling ghee and oil and with flames of circular motion, he would not become pure.

Fish stay in the sacred Ganges and other rivers. Flocks of birds stay in the temples. But they do not attain any special benefit from the ceremonial ablutions and charitable gifts because they are devoid of sacred feelings.

It is the purity of the feelings that is the mark of sanctity of rites.

A person can get caught up in emotions, and a person can rid himself of base emotions. A person purified by pure emotions attains heaven and then liberation.

Shiva-Purāna

Overcoming Depression

*Depression is a thief entering the body. It arises from
ignorance. When that disappears through spiritual
opening (*unmesha*), then, in the absence of a cause,
how can depression remain?*

"Depression in the body" means the dwindling of
delight of the person who is deluded by the body. The
"thief" is that which steals the treasure of Consciousness (*samvid*) and causes the poverty of limitation, and
so on. The origination, or creation, and the continua-
tion of that depression are due to ignorance, that is, to a
failure to recognize that one's essential nature is a Mass
of Consciousness-Bliss. . . . In the absence of depression,
such conditions as sickness, as well as states of torment,
are necessarily eliminated for the yogi. His essential
nature will light up accordingly, like highly heated gold
when the dross is removed. Thus the glory of a great
yogi abiding in the body is the constant absence of
depression. As the great *yoginī* Madālasā, instructing
her young children, said:

*Don't commit the foolishness of thinking that you
are in the body, which is a mere decaying covering to*

be abandoned. Like a jacket, this body clings to you
because of your auspicious and inauspicious deeds,
your delusion, and so forth.

Spanda-Kārikā with *Spanda-Nirnaya*

Give Up Pride

Kabīr, be not proud of your body—
 A sheet of skin stuffed with bones;
They who rode stately horses
 Under canopies of gold
Now lie wrapped in earth.

Kabīr, be not proud
 Of your lofty mansions:
Today or tomorrow
 The earth will be your bed
And grass will cover your head.

Kabīr, be not proud
 Nor sneer at the forlorn;
Your canoe is still in the sea,
 Who knows what its fate will be?

Kabīr, be not proud
 Of your beauty and youth;
This day or the next
 You will have to leave it,
Like a serpent its slough.

KABĪR

Humility

The Lord loves humility first of all. It behooves you, therefore, to do that which will induce humility. The society of the saints is the best place to develop it. The company of priests and pandits who care for nothing else but wealth and good food will not develop humility, nor will the Lord be pleased. Whoever is eager to develop this quality should first seek a living true guru (*sad-guru*) and devote himself to him.

—*Sār Bachan*

Nonviolence

Ahimsā (nonviolence) is the highest ideal. It is meant for the brave, never for the cowardly. . . . No power on earth can subjugate you when you are armed with the sword of *ahimsā*. It ennobles both the victor and the vanquished.

GANDHI

The Do's and Don'ts of
Spiritual Life

❦

Sage Nārada said:

Truthfulness, compassion, austerity, purity, forbearance, tranquillity, self-control, nonharming, chastity, renunciation, study, rectitude,

contentment, serving with equal vision, gradual nonparticipation in village-related activities, consideration of what are wrong activities for people, silence, self-examination,

appropriate distribution of food and so on to beings, and, O Pāndava, regarding them as oneself or as divinity, as well as

listening to the scriptures, praising Him, remembering the greatness of the path, devotional service, worship, humility, servitude to the Lord, friendship, and self-surrender:

These are described as the preeminent duty (*dharma*) for all human beings. He who has these thirty characteristics, O King, is pleasing to the Great Self.

Bhāgavata-Purāna

Life Is a Test

There are various tests to which a devotee is subjected: they could be of the mind, of the intellect, of the body, and so on. . . . In fact God is conducting tests all the time; every occurrence in life is a test. Every thought that crops up in the mind is in itself a test to see what one's reaction will be. Hence one must be always alert and aloof, conducting oneself with a spirit of detachment, viewing everything as an opportunity afforded to gain experience, to improve oneself and go on to a higher stage.

BHAGAWAN NITYANANDA

Inner Transformation

❀

Look here—we shall all die! Bear this in mind always, and then the spirit within will wake up. Then, only, meanness will vanish from you, practicality in work will come, you will get new vigor in mind and body, and those who come in contact with you will also feel that they have really got something uplifting, from you. . . . At first, the heart will break down, and despondency and gloomy thoughts will occupy your mind. But persist, let days pass like that—and then? Then you will see that new strength has come into the heart, that the constant thought of death is giving you new life, and is making you more and more thoughtful by bringing every moment before your mind's eye the truth of the saying, "Vanity of vanities, all is vanity." Wait! Let days, months and years pass, and you will feel that the spirit within is waking up with the strength of a lion, that the little power within has transformed itself into a mighty power!

SWAMI VIVEKANANDA

Ripe and Unripe Beings

Embodied beings are said to be twofold: ripe and unripe.

Unripe embodied beings lack Yoga; the ripe ones are with Yoga. Through the fire of Yoga, the entire body is rendered sentient and free from grief.

However, the unripe body should be understood to be insentient, earthen, and bestowing suffering.

Yoga-Shikhā-Upanishad

Control of Impulses

Hamsa said:

The impulse of speech, the mental impulse of anger,
the impulse of knowledge, and the impulses of belly
and sex organ—I deem him who conquers all these
impulses to be a brahmin and a sage.

Freedom from anger is better than anger. Likewise
being patient is better than being impatient. Manliness
is better than unmanliness. A knowledgeable person is
superior to an ignoramus.

When angry one should not yell furiously. By being
patient, one burns the assailant's good karma (*sukrita*)
and creates it for oneself.

Mahābhārata

Silence

Sage Vasishtha said:

O Rāma, the finest of sages say there are two kinds of sage (*muni*). The first is the severe ascetic; the other is one who is liberated while still alive.

The sage practicing severe asceticism has forcibly conquered the senses. He is undoubtedly bound to arid, nonmeditative rituals.

He who has realized this world as it really is [i.e., as the Self], is well contented, regards the world as before [i.e., like a dream], and is established in the Self by means of the contemplated Self is known as a liberated sage.

The behavior of these two types of peaceful master sages, which has the essential nature of mental resoluteness, is described by the word "silence" (*mauna*).

People knowledgeable about silence say that there are four varieties: silence of speech, silence of the eye, severe silence, and the silence of sleep.

Silence of speech is the control of one's utterances. Silence of the eye is the forceful restraint of the senses. What is known as severe silence consists in abandoning activities.

One who is liberated while still alive practices the silence of sleep in the state of enlightenment. Silence of the mind, which occurs upon death or in severe asceticism, is a fifth kind [and is significantly different from the silence of one who is liberated while still alive].

Yoga-Vāsishtha

Truthfulness

Into those who are truthful,
He merges in truth.
But He never appears
to those who are untruthful.
At the end of time,
He stands as the Lord
accomplishing the liberation of all.
Those who are truthful
come to sport in true joy.

He is united with those
who are united in truth.
He is the pure one
who does not enter false hearts.
When the life force ascends
in the central channel (*sushumnā*)
and you meet the Lord,
then He will abide
in your thoughts.

When thus He abides
in your thoughts,

contemplate Him day and night.
Then He will manifest
above the head.
And if you abandon falsehood
and worldly desires,
the Lord reveals Himself to you
in truth.

Whether or not you reach
the pinnacle of Yoga
is God's grace.
Such is the way of salvation
taught by the great Nandi.
If you subdue the nine deceptive senses,
you may well mount the steed of truth.

Nandi, who has entered
my central channel
and is ever in my thoughts
and inhabits my body:
He is the Blessed One,
the source of all the Vedas,
who does not reveal Himself
to those who are untruthful.
He is the refuge only of those
who shed falsehood.

Tiru-Mandiram

The Nature of Truth

There is no virtue greater than truth; there is no sin greater than falsehood. Therefore a mortal being should take refuge in truth with his entire self.

Worship without truth is worthless; recitation (*japa*) without truth is worthless; asceticism (*tapas*) without truth is likewise worthless—like planting seed in salty earth.

The nature of truth is the supreme Absolute. Truth is the most excellent asceticism. All actions are rooted in truth. Nothing is superior to truth.

Mahānirvāna-Tantra

Three Kinds of Giving

The gift that is given because it ought to be given to a worthy recipient for no reward at the proper place and right time is held to be *sattva*-natured.

The gift that is given reluctantly and with the view of reward, or that aims at the fruit in the afterlife, is held to be *rajas*-natured.

The gift that is given at the wrong place and time to an unworthy recipient, or is given unkindly and contemptuously, is called *tamas*-natured.

Bhagavad-Gītā

Solitude

Worldlings should shun solitude (*ekākitva*) because of their fear, laziness, and so on. They should seek out the company of people, as there is no susceptibility in this. In the case of yogis, however, the opposite is true. The whole of space appears filled with the Self's supreme bliss by means of their continuing meditation in solitude. Hence they are not prone to fear, laziness, sorrow, delusion, and the like.

> *How can there be delusion or sorrow for one who, perceiving only singularity, knows all beings as his very Self?* [Īsha-Upanishad 7]

Thus declares the revealed tradition (*shruti*). A densely populated place is adverse to meditation because of political discussion, and so forth. Therefore it is not conducive to approaching the Self's bliss. Rather, it troubles the mind that seemingly lacks such bliss. The reason for this is the illusoriness of the world and the fullness of the Self.

Jīovanmukti-Viveka

Always Serve Others

The salt of life is selfless service. The bread of life is universal love. Life is not fully lived, life has not been fully realised, if you do not serve and love the entire humanity. The secret of true life is in the love of God and the service of humanity. Live to help others. The divine power will stream through you as a life-giving force.

Swami Sivananda

Worship with the Body

With your whole body as a rosary
Take the name of the Compassionate:
Let this be your worship;
Your fast, acknowledgment of the One,
Putting from you every other;
Your creed, the confession of the Self alone.

DĀDŪ

True Worship

Whether one has bathed or has not taken a bath, or whether one is fasting or eating, one should always worship the supreme Self with a pure mind.

Mahānirvāna-Tantra

The Liberating Power of Devotion

Lord Krishna said:

Those I deem most disciplined who, fixing their mind on Me, always worship Me with good discipline and supreme faith.

But those who worship the imperishable, indefinable Unmanifest, omnipresent, unthinkable, summit-abiding, unmoving, and stable,

and who, restraining the hosts of the senses and the higher mind (*buddhi*) and while remaining the same in everything, take delight in the welfare of all beings—they attain Me.

Greater is the struggle of those whose mind clings to the Unmanifest, for the Unmanifest is reached by embodied beings through a sorrowful course.

But those who have renounced their actions in Me, are intent on Me and none other—they worship Me by contemplating Me through Yoga.

Those whose mind is fixed on Me, O Son of Prithā, I will before long lift out of the death cycle (*mrityu-samsāra*).

Place your mind in Me alone. Let your higher mind settle down in Me. Henceforth you shall dwell in Me alone. Of this there is no doubt.

The yogi who is ever contented, self-controlled, of firm resolve, with his mind and higher mind offered up in Me, who is My devotee—he is dear to Me.

Renouncing in thought all actions to Me, intent on Me, resorting to the Yoga of the higher mind (*buddhi-yoga*), be constantly Me-minded.

Me-minded, you will transcend all obstacles by My grace. But if out of ego sense (*ahamkāra*) you will not listen, then you will perish.

Fully relinquishing all duties (*dharma*), go to Me alone for shelter. I will deliver you from all sin. Do not grieve!

Bhagavad-Gītā

The Path of Devotion

Sage Nārada said:

The radical (*ekāntin*) devotees are foremost.

Conversing with each other with choking throat and tears of ecstasy, they purify their families and the Earth.

They render sacred places (*tīrtha*) sacred; they render actions right; they endow scriptures with true meaning.

They are filled with Him.

The ancestors rejoice; the gods dance, and this Earth obtains a protector.

In them there is no distinction of birth, knowledge, beauty, family, wealth, profession, and so forth.

Bhakti-Sūtra

Mad with Love

I am mad with love
And no one understands my plight.
Only the wounded
Understand the agonies of the wounded,
When a fire rages in the heart.
Only the jeweler knows the value of a jewel,
Not the one who lets it go.
In pain I wandered from door to door,
But could not find a doctor.
Says Mīrā: Harken, my Master,
Mīrā's pain will subside
When Shyām comes as the doctor.

Without my beloved Master
I cannot live.
Body, mind, and life   .
Have I given to the Beloved.
Fascinated by His beauty,
I gaze down the road
Night and day.
Says Mīrā: My Lord, accept your servant—
It is all she asks.

MĪRĀBĀĪ

Love Is the Self

Questioner: Love postulates duality. How can the Self be the object of love?

Ramana Maharshi: Love is not different from the Self. Love of an object is of a lower type and cannot endure, whereas the Self is Love. God is love.

Talks with Sri Ramana Maharshi

The Yoga of Tears

Weep at least once to see God.

SRI RAMAKRISHNA

The Road to Heaven Is through Hell

If there is any road to Heaven, it is through Hell. Through Hell to Heaven is always the way. When the soul has wrestled with circumstance and has met death, a thousand times death on the way, but nothing daunted has struggled forward again and again and yet again—then the soul comes out as a giant and laughs at the ideal he has been struggling for, because he finds how much greater is he than the ideal.

SWAMI VIVEKANANDA

How to Overcome Defects

Faults should be burned off by breath control,
guilt by concentration, addictions by resistance,
and unlorldly qualities by meditation.

Manu-Smriti

Real Fasting

Questioner: Can fasting help realization?

Ramana Maharshi: Yes, but it is only a temporary help. Mental fasting is the real aid. Fasting is not an end in itself. There must be spiritual development at the same time. Absolute fasting weakens the mind too and leaves you without sufficient strength for the spiritual quest. Therefore eat in moderation and go on practicing.

Talks with Sri Ramana Maharshi

The Best Posture

Questioner: There are several *āsanas* (postures) mentioned. Which of them is the best?

Ramana Maharshi: Nididhyāsana (one-pointedness of the mind) is the best posture.

Talks with Sri Ramana Maharshi

The Life Force

The Lord said:

The life force (*prāna*) verily is one's greatest friend; the life force verily is one's greatest companion. O beautiful one, there is no greater kinsman than the life force; indeed there is none.

Shiva-Svarodaya

Breath Control

❀

Sage Vasishtha said:

When the energy of the life force (*prāna*) is restricted,
O Rāma, then the mind dissolves, like the shadow of a
thing when the thing is absent. The mind is of the form
of the life force.

The life force knows one's experience of other places
that are fixed in one's heart. The mind is explained to
be that which stems from the experience of vibration
(*spanda*).

The currents of the life force are restrained through
dispassion, the practice of philosophical argument,
reasoning, and the abstention of effort, as well as
knowledge of the ultimate Reality.

The energy of a rock has mobility like fuel but is not
mental. Energy exists by virtue of vibration.

Vibration is the energy of the currents of the life force, which appears dynamic but is insentient. The energy of consciousness of the Self is transparent and ever praised by all.

The mind is considered to be the union of the energy of consciousness and the energy of vibration. This is said to be false knowledge arising from misconception.

This is called ignorance and it is also labeled illusion (*māyā*). This great ignorance of It produces the poison of the world of change, and so forth.

The conjunction of the energy of consciousness and the energy of vibration with the volition and imagination leads to the creation of the terrors of existence unless volition and imagination are checked.

When the mind thinks, the energy of vibration is caused by the breath (*vāyu*), and then the mind causes thinking of thoughts, including thoughts about the deities, and volitions, and so on.

Yoga-Vāsishtha

Restraining the Senses

Whatever he perceives with his eyes, that he should
    contemplate as being within himself.
Whatever he smells with his nose, that he should
    contemplate as being within himself.
Whatever he tastes with his tongue, that he should
    contemplate as being within himself.
Whatever he touches with his skin, that he should
    contemplate as being within himself.
Thus the yogi should, every day for one *yāma* [three
    hours] without laxity, endeavor
to pull together the many objects of the cognitive
    senses.

Yoga-Shāstra

Recitation Only

The Lord said:

There is no sacrifice greater than the sacrifice of recitation (*japa*). There is nothing greater than that in this world. Therefore one should cultivate virtue, prosperity, cultural enjoyment (*kāma*), and liberation by means of recitation.

Abandoning all other means, one should practice mantric verses. From attentiveness comes success. The fruit of heedlessness is inauspicious.

Recitation is auspicious insofar as it contains a kind of vow to intend the end of worldly enjoyment. Therefore, O Goddess, one should practice Yoga consisting of recitation and meditation.

O Beloved, blemishes resulting from one's transgression of the disciplines—from the individual (*jīva*) to Brahma—done knowingly or unknowingly are removed through recitation.

Kula-Arnava-Tantra

Successful Mantra Practice

※

Questioner: While making *nāma-japa* [recitation of the divine Name] for an hour or more I fall into a state like sleep. On waking up I recollect that my invocation has been interrupted, so I try again.

Ramana Maharshi: "Like sleep," that is right. It is the natural state. Because you are now associated with the ego, you consider that the natural state is something which interrupts your work. So you must have the experience repeated until you realize that it is your natural state. You will then find that *japa* is extraneous but still it will go on automatically. Your present doubt is due to false identity, namely that of identifying yourself with the mind that does the *japa*. *Japa* means clinging to one thought to the exclusion of all others. That is the purpose of it. It leads to *dhyana* [meditation], which ends in Self-realization or *jnāna*.

The Spiritual Teaching of Ramana Maharshi

The Pleasing Inner Sound

❀

Like a bee drinking the nectar is unaware of the scent, so the mind that is ever attached to the inner sound (*nāda*) does not desire any other object.

Bound by the fragrance of the pleasing inner sound, it swiftly abandons its fickleness. Held by the inner sound, the mind—like a snake abiding in the hollow of the body—

forgets the world, becomes one-pointed, and stops running in every direction. For the mad elephant of the mind, roaming in the pleasure garden of worldly objects,

the inner sound is a sharp hook that has the purpose of control. The inner sound is a snare that serves to trap the deer within.

And it is a dam that serves to restrict the inner waves.

Nāda-Upanishad

Concentration

The mind is a thing that dwells in diffusion, in succession; it can only concentrate on one thing at a time and when not concentrated runs from one thing to another very much at random. Therefore it has to concentrate on a single idea, a single subject of meditation, a single object of contemplation, a single object of will in order to possess or master it, and this it must do to at least the temporary exclusion of all others. But that which is beyond the mind and into which we seek to rise is superior to the running process of the thought, superior to the division of ideas. The Divine is centred in itself and when it throws out ideas and activities does not divide itself or imprison itself in them, but holds them and their movement in its infinity; undivided, its whole self is behind each Idea and each movement and at the same time behind all of them together. Held by it, each spontaneously works itself out, not through a separate act of will, but by the general force of consciousness behind it; if to us there seems to be a concentration of divine Will and Knowledge in each, it is a multiple and equal and not an exclusive concentration, and the reality of it is rather a free and spontaneous working in a self-gathered unity and infinity. The soul which has risen to the divine Samadhi [ecstatic concentration] participates in the measure of its attainment in this reversed condition of things—the true condition, for that which is the reverse of our mentality is the truth. It is for this reason that, as is said in the ancient books, the man who has arrived at Self-possession attains spontaneously without the need of concentration in thought and effort the knowledge or the result which the Idea or the Will in him moves out to embrace.

To arrive then at this settled divine status must be the object of our concentration. The first step in concentration must be always to accustom the discursive mind to a settled unwavering pursuit of a single course of connected thought on a single subject and this it must do undistracted by all lures and alien calls on its attention. Such concentration is common enough in our ordinary life, but it becomes more difficult when we have to do it inwardly without any outward object or action on which to keep the mind; yet this inward concentration is what the seeker of knowledge must effect. Nor must it be merely the consecutive thought of the intellectual thinker, whose only object is to conceive and intellectually link together his conceptions. It is not, except perhaps at first, a process of reasoning that is wanted so much as a dwelling so far as possible on the fruitful essence of the idea which by the insistence of the soul's will upon it must yield up all the facets of its truth.

SRI AUROBINDO

Be the Observer

❀

Question: Everybody says: "I work, I come, I go."

Sri Nisargadatta Maharaj: I have no objection to the conventions of your language, but they distort and destroy reality. A more accurate way of saying would have been: "There is talking, working, coming, going." For anything to happen, the entire universe must coincide. It is wrong to believe that anything in particular can cause an event. Every cause is universal. Your very body would not exist without the entire universe contributing to its creation and survival. I am fully aware that things happen as they happen because the world is as it is. To affect the course of events I must bring a new factor into the world and such factor can only be myself, the power of love and understanding focused in me.

When the body is born, all kinds of things happen to it and you take part in them because you take yourself to be the body. You are like the man in the cinema, laughing and crying with the picture though knowing fully well that he is all the time in his seat and the picture is but the play of light. It is enough to shift attention from the screen to oneself to break the spell. When the body dies, the kind of life you live now—succession of physical and mental events—comes to an end. It can end even now—without waiting for the death of the body—it is enough to shift attention to the self and keep it there. All happens as if there is a mysterious power that creates and moves everything. Realize that you are not the mover, only the observer, and you will be at peace.

Question: Is that power separate from me?

Maharaj: Of course not. But you must begin by being the dispassionate observer. Then only will you realise your full being as the universal lover and actor. As long as you are enmeshed in the tribulations of a particular personality, you can see nothing beyond it. But ultimately you will come to see that you are neither the particular nor the universal, you are beyond both. As a tiny point of the pencil can draw innumerable pictures so does the dimensionless point of awareness draw the contents of the vast universe. Find that point and be free.

I Am That

The Greatest Work

One should contemplate oneself *as* the world. For him who contemplates himself as the world, his work is not exhausted, because out of himself he creates whatever he desires.

Brihad-Āranyaka-Upanishad

Transform the World through Meditation

❀

If you made a sweet pudding, full of delicious ingredients—pistachios, almonds, cardamon—but left out the sugar, how could it have any taste? In the same way, the world can be enjoyable only if you meditate on God. Through meditation man can make the world his greatest friend; without meditation on God, the world is full of suffering and pain. The truth is that life in the world can be a magnificent way to happiness, but only if God is in it completely. Without remembrance of God, without knowledge of Him, without meditation on Him, worldly life is crippled; it has no savor, no delight.

Don't abandon the world and your near and dear ones. Don't waste your strength running in every direction in search of God. Don't lose yourself while you look for peace and rest. Beloved people, stay at home with your husbands, your wives, your children. Be friendly with your crafts, skills, and talents. Stay with your businesses and factories. According to destiny, you may be a rich man or a laborer, a king or a beggar, but God belongs to everyone.

SWAMI MUKTANANDA

Obstacles to Meditation

❧

Sickness, languor, doubt, heedlessness, sloth, dissipa-
tion, false vision, and nonattainment of the stages of
meditation and instability in them are the distractions
of the mind; these are the obstacles.

There are nine obstacles or distractions of the mind
(*citta*). These appear together with the fluctuations of
the mind. They are not found in the absence of the pre-
viously mentioned fluctuations of the mind [i.e., correct
perception, erroneous perception, conceptualization,
memory, and sleep]. Of these, sickness is a disorder of
the humors, the secretions, or the organs. Languor is a
lack of activity of the mind. Doubt is thinking that
touches alternatives, such as "This might be so or this
might not be so." Heedlessness is not cultivating the
means of ecstasy (*samādhi*). Sloth is inactivity due to
heaviness of the body or the mind. Dissipation is mental
greed consisting in addiction to the sense objects. False
vision is false knowledge. Nonattainment of a stage is
nonattainment of any stage of ecstasy. Instability is the
mind's inability to remain in a stage once it has been
attained. If a stage of ecstasy had actually been attained,

the mind would of course have remained in it. Thus these mental distractions are called the nine blemishes of Yoga, the foes of Yoga, or the obstacles to Yoga.

Pain, depression, bodily tremor, wrong inhalation,
and wrong exhalation accompany the distractions.

Pain originating in oneself, pain originating from other beings, and pain originating from the deities—all pain is that by which living beings are stricken down and for the removal of which they struggle. Depression is agitation of the mind due to an impediment caused by a desire. Tremor of the body is that which makes the limbs tremble and shake. Inhalation is breathing that sucks in the outside air. Exhalation is that which causes the abdominal air to flow outward. These are the accompaniments of the distractions. They occur in a distracted mind but do not occur in a focused mind.

To countermand these, one should practice with
regard to a single principle.

To countermand these distractions, one should train the mind to rest upon a single principle.

Yoga-Sūtra with *Yoga-Bhāshya*

Ecstasy

Just as salt dissolves in water, so, for the knower of Yoga, the mind and the Self become identical: this is described as ecstasy (*samādhi*).

There is also another view:

That state in which the individual self and the transcendental Self are in equilibrium (*samatva*) and in which all concepts are transcended is described as ecstasy.

Hatha-Ratna-Avalī

Pathway to Ecstasy

Ecstasy is the supreme Yoga, which is attained by great fortune, the teacher's compassion and grace, and by devotion to the teacher.

The yogi who, day after day, cultivates confidence in the transmitted knowledge, confidence in the teacher, and self-confidence quickly reaches the very auspicious practice of ecstasy.

Separating the mind from the "pot" [i.e., the body], one should unite it with the transcendental Self. By freeing oneself from attachment to the ten conditions, one should know that ecstasy.

Gheranda-Samhitā

Psychic Powers

Powers (*siddhi*) are twofold in this world: artificial and nonartificial.

Those powers that are perfected by means of alchemical potions, herbs, ritual, magic, and the repetition of mantras are known as artificial.

Powers produced by external means are merely temporary and have little energy. But those not generated by external means come about spontaneously

in those who are dedicated solely to the Yoga of their innate Self. These powers are numerous and dear to the Primal Lord and are known as devoid of artifice.

They are accomplished, permanent, highly energetic, and manifest after a long time in those free from traits (*vāsanā*), as a result of their Yoga and in compliance with their will.

He who, by the great Yoga, resides in the eternal abode of the supreme Self should keep them secret. The characteristic abilities of a Yoga adept must be kept secret unless they have to be deployed for the benefit of others.

Just as pilgrims on the way to Kāshī (Banaras) see various holy places, and as accomplishments in various paths

arise of their own accord, so those on the path of Yoga who are free from concern for loss or gain encounter a range of powers.

Just as assaying goldsmiths identify gold, so one can recognize an adept who is liberated while still alive by his powers.

To be sure, the quality of "otherworldliness" will sometimes be seen in him. One should consider a man lacking in powers as being bound.

Yoga-Shikhā-Upanishad

The Seven Stages of Wisdom

❀

At first one should develop wisdom in association with tradition (*shāstra*) and holy folk. This is said to be the first stage of Yoga of the nine yogis.

The second is inquiry. The third is the cultivation of nonattachment. The fourth is eradication, consisting in the removal of the traits (*vāsanā*).

That which manifests as the bliss of pure Consciousness is the fifth. Herein abides he who is liberated in life, who shines forth fully awake even when half asleep.

That which manifests as nonexperience is the sixth stage, which is formed by a single mass of bliss and is a state corresponding to deep sleep.

The auspicious seventh stage, transcending the Fourth State, alone is liberation, which consists in sameness and transparency.

Laghu-Yoga-Vāsishta

The Self Is the Foundation of All

As the ocean is the single locus of all waters,
as the skin is the single locus of all touch,
as the nostrils are the single locus of all smells,
as the tongue is the single locus of all tastes,
as the eye is the single locus of all forms,
as the ear is the single locus of all sounds,
as the mind is the single locus of all ideas,
as the heart is the single locus of all knowledge,
as the hands are the single locus of all acts,
as the genitals are the single locus of all pleasure,
as the feet are the single locus of all movement,
as the speech is the single locus of all the Vedas
—thus is That [i.e., the Self].

As a lump of salt, when thrown in water,
dissolves in water, and no one can perceive it,
because from wherever one takes it, it tastes salty
—thus, my dear, this great, endless, transcendental
    Being
is but a Mass of Awareness (*vijñāna-ghana*).

Brihad-Āranyaka-Upanishad

For the Sake of the Self

Sage Yājnavalkya said:

Verily, not for the sake of the husband is the husband dear but for the sake of the Self is the husband dear. Verily, not for the sake of the wife is the wife dear but for the sake of the Self is the wife dear. Verily, not for the sake of one's sons are one's sons dear but for the sake of the Self are one's sons dear. Verily, not for the sake of wealth is wealth dear but for the sake of the Self is wealth dear. . . . Verily, not for the sake of everything is everything dear but for the sake of the Self is everything dear. Verily, O Maitreyi, the Self should be seen, heard, thought about, meditated upon. Indeed, upon seeing, hearing, thinking about, and knowing the Self, all this is known.

Brihad-Āranyaka-Upanishad

The Immortal Inner Controller

❀

Sage Uddālaka Āruni said:

He who dwells in all beings and is within all beings,
whom all beings do not know, whose body is all
beings, who controls all beings from within—he is the
Self (*ātman*), the immortal inner controller
(*antaryāmin*). Thus it is relative to beings; relative to
the self.

He who dwells in the life force (*prāna*) and is within
the life force, whom the life force does not know,
whose body is the life force, who guides the life force
from within—he is the Self, the immortal inner controller.

He who dwells in the organ of speech and is within the
organ of speech, whom the organ of speech does not
know, whose body is the organ of speech, who controls
the organ of speech from within—he is the Self, the
immortal inner controller.

He who dwells in the eye and is within the eye, whom

the eye does not know, whose body is the eye, who controls the eye from within—he is the Self, the immortal inner controller.

He who dwells in the ear and is within the ear, whom the ear does not know, whose body is the ear, who controls the ear from within—he is the Self, the immortal inner controller.

He who dwells in the mind (*manas*) and is within the mind, whom the mind does not know, whose body is the mind, who controls the mind from within—he is the Self, the immortal inner controller.

He who dwells in the skin and is within the skin, whom the skin does not know, whose body is the skin, who controls the skin from within—he is the Self, the immortal inner controller.

He who dwells in understanding and is within understanding, whom understanding does not know, whose body is understanding, who controls understanding from within—he is the Self, the immortal inner controller.

He who dwells in semen and is within semen, whom semen does not know, whose body is semen, who controls semen from within—he is the Self, the immortal inner controller. He is the unseen Seer, the unheard

Hearer, the unthought Thinker, the not-understood Understander. There is no other Seer than he. There is no other Hearer than he. There is no other Thinker than he. There is no other Understander than he. He is the Self, the immortal inner controller. What is other than that is afflicted. Thereafter Uddālaka Āruni fell silent.

Brihad-Āranyaka-Upanishad

The Serpent Power Awakens

Suddenly, with a roar like that of a waterfall, I felt a stream of liquid light entering my brain through the spinal cord.

Entirely unprepared for such a development, I was completely taken by surprise; but regaining self-control instantaneously, I remained sitting in the same posture, keeping my mind on the point of concentration. The illumination grew brighter and brighter, the roaring louder, I experienced a rocking sensation and then felt myself slipping out of my body, entirely enveloped in a halo of light. It is impossible to describe the experience accurately. I felt the point of consciousness that was myself growing wider, surrounded by waves of light. It grew wider and wider, spreading outward while the body, normally the immediate object of its perception, appeared to have receded into the distance until I became entirely unconscious of it. I was now all consciousness, without any outline, without any idea of a corporeal appendage, without any feeling or sensation coming from the senses, immersed in a sea of light simultaneously conscious and aware of every point, spread out, as it were, in all directions without any barrier or material obstruction.

GOPI KRISHNA

The Long-Haired Ascetic

The long-haired one (*keshin*) bears fire;
the long-haired one bears poison;
the long-haired one bears the world;
the long-haired one gazes fully on heaven;
the long-haired one is said to be that Light.

The wind-girt sages have donned the tawny dust.
Along the wind's course they glide
when the Gods have penetrated them.

Exulted by our silence,
upon the winds we have ascended.
Of us, O mortals, you behold only our bodies.

Through the middle space (*antariksha*) flies the sage
shining down upon all forms.
For his goodness, he is deemed the friend of every God.

The wind's steed, Vāyu's friend,
is the God-intoxicated sage.
He dwells within both oceans, upper and lower.

Along the paths of fairies, elves, and beasts
wanders the long-haired one,
knower of thoughts, a most exhilarating, gentle friend.

For him Vāyu has churned and pounded the unbendable,
when the long-haired one drank with Rudra from the
   poison cup.

Rig-Veda

Floating in the Divine

૱

After crossing the seven rings of light of the central region [of divine existence], one enters the vast and limitless expanse, the Infinite, and starts swimming in it. Here the guru's assistance is still needed, since even the subtlest force of the swimmer in the act of his heavy swimming sets up waves of energy that erect a barrier against progress. Only the experienced, capable and watchful guru helps in settling the waves and teaching the swimmer the art of light swimming which is almost akin to floating but still is not floating, which type of swimming does not set up opposing waves. The guru also helps to keep the swimmer from slipping into enjoyment of the state of light swimming which will impede further progress, and takes him on the further journey.

Now we reach the sphere of the dormant Centre which also seems to be enclosed by something like a ring, which is the last. For the sake of expression and experiment, I once made an attempt to enter into it; but a sudden, strong and forceful push threw me back, though I was able to get a moment's peep into it. This has made me conclude that this is perhaps the last possible limit of human approach . . . Here we are in close harmony with the very Real condition.

RAM CHANDRA

Embodied Liberation

After millions of years and thousands of births, he arrives at the shore of Self-realization.

Thus all means to the end come naturally to him, and he sits on the very throne of discrimination.

Then with the speed of thought itself even discrimination is left behind, and he becomes one with that which is beyond thought.

The cloud in the form of the mind vanishes; the air loses its very nature and is absorbed into itself.

He enjoys indescribable bliss, such that the sacred syllable (*om*) lowers its head, and language retreats before him.

Thus he becomes the embodiment of the state of Brahma, that which promotes all activity, and is indeed the very form of the Formless.

During many past lives he has swept away the mass of confusion, and the moment of his birth is the final moment of his marriage [with Brahma],

and entering into nonduality he becomes wedded with the Eternal, as the clouds merge into the sky.

So while still in the body, he becomes one with the Eternal, from which the universe proceeds and into which it will again be absorbed.

Jnāneshvarī

The Liberated Sage

Even though one may be engaged in worldly activity, he whose mind, whether inactive or active, abides like space itself—he is said to be liberated while still alive.

He whose mental radiance does not rise or set in happiness or suffering and who remains the same in whatever condition he meets—he is said to be liberated while still alive.

He who is wakeful while asleep, who knows no waking, whose waking is free from desires—he is said to be liberated while still alive.

He who, though acting in accord with attachment, aversion, fear, and so on, is as exceedingly transparent as the inner space—he is said to be liberated while still alive.

He whose mental state is not affected by ego and whose higher mind is not tainted, whether he is active or passive—he is said to be liberated while still alive.

He from whom the world does not recoil and who does not recoil from the world, who is released from joy, anger, and fear—he is said to be liberated while still alive.

He who, though engaging in the web of worldly things, yet remains cool, and who abides as the whole Self amid seemingly other things—he is said to be liberated while still alive.

O sage, when he who is content in Me, the Self of all, gives up all mind-born desires— he is said to be liberated while still alive.

He whose unagitated mind rests in the supremely holy State, pure Consciousness devoid of thoughts—he is said to be liberated while still alive.

He in whose mind thoughts like "I am the world" or "this is He" and the conglomerate of visible phenomena do not burst forth—he is said to be liberated while still alive.

Varāha-Upanishad

The Supreme Swan

Nārada, approaching the Lord, asked: "Now, what is the path of the yogis who are supreme swans (*paramahamsa*), and what is their state?"

The Lord said to him: "The path of the supreme swans is most difficult to find in this world. There are not many, but even if there is only one of them, he abides in that which is ever pure; he indeed is the man of the Vedas. Thus think the sages. This great man has his mind always abide in Me, and therefore I abide in him as well. Renouncing his own sons, wife, relatives, friends, and so on, and giving up his hair tuft, sacrificial thread, study, and all works, as well as the world at large, he should take up a staff, loincloth, and other covering for the maintenance of his body and for the good of the world. But this is not of foremost importance. If asked what is foremost, it is this:

"The supreme swan does not carry a staff, tuft, sacrificial thread, and covering. He knows neither cold nor heat, neither pleasure nor pain, neither honor nor dishonor. He is beyond the six waves [of the world ocean, namely, hunger, thirst, grief, delusion, decrepitude, and death] by giving up censure, pride, jealousy, deceitfulness, haughtiness, longing, hatred, pleasure, pain, desire, anger, greed, delusion, elation, envy, egoism, and so on. He looks upon his own body as a corpse, because the body's degradation is the cause of doubt, perversity, and erroneous knowledge. Always turning away from the world and always understanding That, he enters that state himself. 'I am that peaceful, immutable, nondual, blissful Mass of Consciousness. That alone is my supreme Home; that alone is my tuft; that alone is my sacrificial thread.' Through knowledge of the unity of the self and the supreme Self, the distinction between them vanishes. This is the dawn [of true gnosis]."

Paramahamsa-Upanishad

How Does the Liberated Sage Behave?

With children, he should behave in a childlike manner. He should be unattached and blameless with the silent pundits. What is called "Aloneness" is the conclusion, gained through cessation of activity. Thus said Prajāpati. Having known the great Abode, one should live under a tree, in rags, unaided, alone, abiding in ecstasy. He who desires the Self has his desires fulfilled and is free from desire, with all desires dwindled. . . . He should be like a tree; when cut down, he does not get angry and does not tremble. He should be like a lotus; when cut down, he does not get angry and does not tremble. He should be like space itself; when cut down, he does not get angry and does not tremble. He should abide with the Truth, for the Truth is the Self.

Subāla-Upanishad

Open-Eyed Ecstasy

Hemalekhā saw that her beloved husband had attained the desired supreme State and did not disturb him. After one *muhūrta* [forty-eight minutes], he awoke from the supreme condition. He opened his eyes and saw his beloved and the surroundings. Eagerly desiring to rest in that condition once more, he closed his eyes. Promptly grasping his hands, she asked her beloved in a beautiful ambrosial voice, "Tell me, what have you found to be the benefit by closing your eyes or the loss by keeping them open? What happens when they are closed? What happens when they are left open? Tell me this, my dearest. I would like to hear about your experience."

Asked in this manner, he said to her, lazily or reluctantly, as if he were drunk on wine or made slow from idleness, "My dear, I have at last found complete repose. I find no rest in external things, which are filled with suffering. Enough of activities, which are like constantly chewing cattle. He who is blinded by misfortune, which lies outside oneself, does not know true joy within himself. Just as someone goes begging for food because he does not know about his own treasure, so did I, ignorant of the ocean of joy within myself, again and again go after the pleasure obtained from things as if they were most excellent, even though they are overflowing with massive suffering and are transient like lightning. I deemed them permanent by force of habit. He who is stricken with suffering does not attain repose. Therefore people unable to distinguish between joy and sorrow always uselessly accumulate a mass of suffering. Enough of such efforts, which merely enhance the experience of suffering. My dear, I beg you with folded hands, be kind to me! I want to find repose in my Self's innate joy again. Oh, you are unfortunate because even though you know this State yourself, you abandon that repose and instead engage in useless activity leading to suffering."

Thus spoken to, the wise woman smiled and said, "My dear, it is you who does not know the supremely holy state, knowing which the learned of pure heart are no longer deluded. That state is as far removed from you as the sky is from the surface of the Earth. What you know is next to nothing. Seeing that state does not depend on closing or opening one's eyes! Nor is it ever attained by doing or not doing something. Nor is that state realized by any coming or going. How can the Whole (*pūrna*) possibly be attained by doing anything, going anywhere, or closing one's eyes? If it were located inside oneself, then how could that state be the Whole? Myriads upon myriads of universes exist in one corner alone. How can these be made to disappear by the mere opening or closing of an eyelid measuring a digit's width? Oh, what can I say about the amazing magnitude of your delusion? Listen, Prince! I will tell you what is the essential truth. So long as the knots of ignorance are not cut, true joy will escape you. There are myriads of knots, which form a rope of delusion. . . . Get rid of the knots and confine the notion 'I perceive' in your heart. Uproot the very tight knot 'I am not this.' Everywhere behold the undivided, blissful, expansive Self. Behold the whole world in the Self, as if it were reflected in a mirror. Do not think that there is more than the Self, which is everywhere and everything. Entering everything, abide as that which also is within by means of the innate Self."

Thus listening to what his beloved said, the brilliant Hemacūda was rid of his misconception and understood that the Self is the Whole, which is everywhere. Gradually he stably realized this by becoming absorbed into the Whole itself and lived forever with Hemalekhā and a host of other maidens.

Tripura-Rahasya

Levels of Bliss

❀

Let there be a youth, a good youth, studied, quick, steady, and strong. Let this entire Earth be filled with wealth for him. That is a single measure of human bliss. One hundred human blisses is a single bliss of human fairies (*gandharva*) and also of one who is versed in the sacred revelation and is not smitten with desire.

One hundred blisses of human fairies is a single bliss of the divine fairies and also of one who is versed in the sacred revelation and is not smitten with desire.

One hundred blisses of divine fairies is a single bliss of the ancestors in their long-enduring world and also of one who is versed in the sacred revelation and is not smitten with desire.

One hundred blisses of the ancestors in their long-enduring world is a single bliss of the deities who are born so by birth and also of one who is versed in the sacred revelation and is not smitten with desire.

One hundred blisses of the deities who are born so by birth is a single bliss of the deities by work, who go to the deities through work and also of one who is versed in the sacred revelation and is not smitten with desire.

One hundred blisses of the deities by work is a single bliss of Indra and also of one who is versed in the sacred revelation and is not smitten with desire.

One hundred blisses of Indra is a single bliss of Brihaspati and also of one who is versed in the sacred revelation and is not smitten with desire.

One hundred blisses of Brihaspati is a single bliss of Prajāpati and also of one who is versed in the sacred revelation and is not smitten with desire.

One hundred blisses of Prajāpati is a single bliss of Brahma and also of one who is versed in the sacred revelation and is not smitten with desire.

He who is here in this person and who is there in the sun—he is One. He who knows thus, upon departing from this world reaches the self made of food, reaches the self made of the life force, reaches the self made of mind, reaches the self made of awareness, reaches the Self made of bliss. On that there also is this verse:

He who knows that bliss of the Absolute (*brahman*) from which words return together with the mind without attaining it fears nothing whatsoever.

Taittirīya-Upanishad

Bliss beyond Pain

My experience is that everything is bliss. But the desire for bliss creates pain. Thus bliss becomes the seed of pain. The entire universe of pain is born of desire. Give up the desire for pleasure and you will not even know what pain is.

NISARGADATTA MAHARAJ

I Am Food

I am food. I am food. I am food.
I am the food eater. I am the food eater. I am the food
 eater.
I am the sound maker. I am the sound maker. I am the
 sound maker.
I am the first-born of the Cosmic Order,
Earlier than the deities, in the navel of immortality.
He who gives me, he indeed saves me.
I, the food, eat the eater of food.
I have overcome the whole world.
I am the brilliant Light.
He who knows thus knows the secret teaching (*upan-
 ishad*).

Taittirīya-Upanishad

Salutation to Myself!

Ah! Me! Salutation to Myself! I do not cease to exist even when the universe is destroyed from Brahma down to a clump of grass.

Ah! Me! Salutation to Myself! Even though I am embodied, I am singular and do not go or come from anywhere but abide pervading the universe.

Ah! Me! Salutation to Myself! No one here is as capable as I who long bear the universe without touching it with the body.

Ah! Me! Salutation to Myself! I have nothing whatsoever and yet have everything that falls within the range of mind and speech.

Ashtāvakra-Samhitā

Cosmic Consciousness

❀

He struck gently on my chest above the heart.

My body became immovably rooted; breath was drawn out of my lungs as if by some huge magnet. Soul and mind instantly lost their physical bondage, and streamed out like a fluid piercing light from my every pore. The flesh was as though dead, yet in my intense awareness I knew that never before had I been fully alive. My sense of identity was no longer narrowly confined to a body, but embraced the circumambient atoms. People on distant streets seemed to be moving gently over my own remote periphery. The roots of plants and trees appeared through a dim transparency of the soil. I discerned the inward flow of their sap.

The whole vicinity lay bare before me. My ordinary frontal vision was now changed to a vast spherical sight, simultaneously all-perceptive. . . .

All objects within my panoramic gaze trembled and vibrated like quick motion pictures. My body, Master's, the pillared courtyard, the furniture and floor, the trees and sunshine, occasionally became violently agitated, until all melted into a luminescent sea; even as sugar crystals, thrown into a glass of water, dissolve after being shaken. The unifying light alternated with materi-alizations of form, the metamorphoses revealing the law of cause and effect in creation.

An oceanic joy broke upon calm endless shores of my soul. The Spirit of God, I realized, is exhaustless Bliss; His body is countless tissues of light. A swelling glory within me began to envelop towns, continents, the earth, solar and stellar systems, tenuous nebulae, and floating universes. The entire cosmos, gently luminous, like a city seen afar at night, glimmered within the infinitude of my being.

PARAMAHAMSA YOGANANDA

I Am He

O Words! Have you the power to describe the ecstatic bliss raging within me? I am blessed. I am really beatified.

It was difficult ever to see clearly the hands, feet, eyes, or ears of the Beloved through the veil or covering (of Maya). How wonderful is it now to behold Him face-to-face with full satisfaction! He is fully exposed to Me. O you bones and flesh of body consciousness! Keep away. O separatism! Go away. O differentiation! Get you gone. Do not come in between us. I am He and He is myself. We are completely united into One. O the ecstatic joy. Why? Why are the tears rolling down at the time of our blissful Union with the Beloved? Are these tears at the death of my mind-consciousness? This is the end of all the worldly rituals. All the desires have faded into nothingness. All the sorrow, sufferings, worries, etc., have disappeared like darkness in light. The armada of evils and virtues is drowned in the vast ocean of Oneness with the Beloved. . . .

How wonderful! I have now discovered and realized that I am Brahman myself. I am myself the Turiya. The One whom we addressed as the third person is Himself the first person. The "third person" is now no more. *It is all One.* There is neither me nor He. Every thing is lost in One. Om! Om!! Om!!!

Swami Rama Tirtha

Immortality

They say that I am dying, but I am not going away.
Where could I go? I am here.

RAMANA MAHARSHI

Sources

ON THE WAY TO THE DIVINE (PAGE 1)
Sri Aurobindo, *The Divine Life* (Pondicherry, India: Sri Aurobindo Ashram, 1977), vol. 1, pp. 42–43. Sri Aurobindo was one of
the truly great philosopher-sages and yogis of the twentieth century. His evolutionary Integral Yoga has caught the attention of
many Western savants and Yoga students.

THE PRECIOUSNESS OF HUMAN EMBODIMENT (PAGES 2–4)
Kula-Arnava-Tantra 1.16–27. Translation by Georg Feuerstein.
The *Kula-Arnava-Tantra*, probably composed in the eleventh or
twelfth century CE, is one of the most important Hindu Tantras.

THE TIME TO REALIZE GOD IS NOW (PAGE 5)
Adapted from the rendering by A. J. Alston in *The Devotional
Poems of Mirabai* (Delhi: Motilal Banarsidass, 1980), p. 117. The
saintly Mīrābāī (1498?–1546 CE), born in Rajasthan, was one of
the great women mystics of the medieval *bhakti* movement. Mar-
ried to the Rajput prince Bhoja at a time of great political turbu-
lence, she knew much human suffering and survived several
attempts on her life, which she attributed to the timely intervention
of the Divine. It appears that later in life, after her husband's
death, she took up the life of a wandering ascetic. The phrase
"beloved Lord" is "Lāl Giridhāra" in the original, which means
"lovely one who upheld the mountain (*giri*)," this being a reference
to Lord Krishna's superhuman feat of holding aloft the entire
Govardhana mountain when a village of devotees was threatened
with extinction from a huge flood.

THE SIGNIFICANCE OF HUMAN LIFE (PAGES 6–7)
Bhāgavata-Purāna 7.6.1–9. Translation by Georg Feuerstein. The *Bhāgavata-Purāna,* also called *Shrīmad-Bhāgavata,* is the most important sacred scripture of the Vaishnavas, the Vishnu worshipers. It was composed in the ninth or tenth century CE and teaches the Yoga of devotion (*bhakti-yoga*). Sage Prahlāda, who speaks the quoted lines, is remembered as one of the great devotees of Vishnu in ancient times.

THE POTENTIAL OF THE BODY (PAGES 8–9)
Yoga-Vāsishtha 4.23.18–24. Translation by Georg Feuerstein. The *Yoga-Vāsishtha* is a didactic work of around thirty thousand stanzas, composed perhaps in the eleventh century CE. Vasishtha (sometimes spelled Vashishtha) is the name of several great adepts of early times. Often later works are attributed to them, as in the present case.

STRENGTHEN THE BODY TO LIBERATE THE MIND (PAGES 10–11)
Gheranda-Samhitā 1.4–8. Translation by Georg Feuerstein. This scripture, written in the late seventeenth century CE, is one of the three principal manuals of *hatha-yoga,* the "forceful Yoga." This Yoga is designed to purify and strengthen the body as a prelude to awakening the serpent power (*kundalinī-shakti*), which is a form of the divine power, or Goddess.

MICROCOSM AND MACROCOSM (PAGE 12)
Shiva-Samhitā 2.1–5. Translation by Georg Feuerstein. This is one of the three fundamental manuals of *hatha-yoga.* It belongs probably to the late seventeenth or early eighteenth century CE. The anonymous author of this text attributes his thoughts to Shiva himself.

THE TRANSMUTED BODY OF THE YOGI (PAGES 13–14)
Yoga-Shikhā-Upanishad 1.38–47. Translation by Georg Feuer-

stein. This Upanishad, probably written in the fifteenth or sixteenth century CE, is one of the so-called *Yoga-Upanishads*, which favor the nondualist metaphysics of Advaita Vedānta.

"I AM THE BODY" IS A LIE (PAGES 15–16)
Tejo-Bindu-Upanishad 5.89–97. Translation by Georg Feuerstein. This Upanishad, one of the *Yoga-Upanishads*, teaches Yoga on the basis of Vedantic nondualism.

FELL THE TREE OF "I" AND "MINE" (PAGES 17–18)
Mārkandeya-Purāna 30.8–13. Translation by Georg Feuerstein. This Purāna is thought to be one of the oldest texts of its genre, perhaps dating from the second or third century CE. Some of its teachings are considerably older, however, having been transmitted by word of mouth for countless generations.

THE WORLD IS ILLUSORY (PAGES 19–20)
Shiva-Samhitā 1.36–39, 62–63. Translation by Georg Feuerstein. About the *Shiva-Samhitā*, see the note to "Microcosm and Macrocosm."

THE FISHING-NET OF THE WORLD (PAGE 21)
Swami Nikhilananda, trans., *The Gospel of Sri Ramakrishna* (New York: Ramakrishna-Vivekananda Center, 1952), pp. 164–65. Sri Ramakrishna (1836–86), the guru of the world-renowned Swami Vivekananda, was one of the great saints of nineteenth-century India. Having his first spiritual experience at the age of six or seven, Ramakrishna attained the state of "formless ecstasy" (*nirvikalpa-samādhi*) in a single day after having been initiated by a Tantric adept. However, he continued to worship the Divine in the form of the goddess Kālī for the rest of his life. The *māyā* of the Divine, mentioned by Ramakrishna, is the creative power by which the world illusion is maintained.

THE UMBRELLA OF MENTAL IMPRESSIONS (PAGE 22)

Meher Baba, *Life at Its Best*, ed. I. O. Duce (New York: Perennial Library, 1972), pp. 35–36. This quote is one of the messages Meher Baba (1894–1969) gave during his visit to the United States in 1956. He taught the gospel of unconditional love (*bhakti*) and was hailed as a divine "descent" (*avatāra*) who, in his own words, "has come not to teach but to awaken."

SUFFERING IS OMNIPRESENT (PAGES 23–24)

Linga-Purāna 1.86.33–35, 37–39. Translation by Georg Feuerstein. This scripture is one of the eighteen major Purānas and was probably composed between the eighth and tenth centuries CE. Its religious orientation is that of Shaivism (centering on the worship of the Divine in the form of Shiva).

THE TRUTH ABOUT JOY AND SORROW (PAGES 25–26)

Mahābhārata 12.168.18–22, 24–25. Translation by Georg Feuerstein. This and all other quotes from the *Mahābhārata* are based on V. S. Sukthankar and S. K. Belvalkar's critical edition of the Sanskrit text. The *Mahābhārata*, which is one of India's two great Sanskrit epics, contains numerous passages expressing yogic teachings, including the celebrated *Bhagavad-Gītā*. The fool mentioned in the passage is happy not because he experiences genuine happiness but because he does not know any better. It is the individuals caught in between the fool and the sage who are really suffering, because they are aware of their unhappiness.

CUTTING THROUGH DESIRE (PAGE 27)

Tiru-Mandiram, 2614–16. Adapted from the translation by B. Natarajan in M. Govindan, ed., *Thirumandiram: A Classic of Yoga and Tantra by Siddhar Thirumoolar* (Montreal: Babaji's Kriya Yoga and Publications, 1993), vol. 3, pp. 8–127. The *Tiru-Mandiram* is a beautiful Tamil work, composed by the adept Tirumūlar, who may have lived in the second century CE. It is a profound Yoga text, though little known in the West.

INSTRUCTION IN HAPPINESS (PAGES 28–31)
Jnāneshvarī 18.770–78, 785–93, 796–98, 802–06. Translation by V. G. Pradhan in H. M. Lambert, ed., *Jnāneshvarī (Bhavārtha-dīpikā)* (London: Allen & Unwin, 1969), vol. 2, pp. 283–85. This extraordinary commentary on the *Bhagavad-Gītā*, written in melodious Marathi, was composed by the adept Jnānadeva (or Jnāneshvara), who was born in 1275 CE and died at the age of twenty-one by entering a deep ecstatic state and voluntarily shedding the body. Thus he appears to have written the *Jnāneshvarī* at an extraordinarily young age.

THE VALUE OF CONTENTMENT (PAGES 32–33)
Bhāgavata-Purāna 7.15.17–25. Translation by Georg Feuerstein. About the *Bhāgavata-Purāna*, see the note to "The Significance of Human Life." The concepts of *sattva* (lucidity, goodness), *rajas* (passion, activity), and *tamas* (dullness, lethargy) are important metaphysical notions of the Yoga and Vedānta traditions. These are the three primary qualities (*guna*) of nature, which keep the world of cyclic existence in perpetual motion. They are both cosmological and psychological factors, and the yogi must learn to master and transcend them through the practice of wisdom-generating meditation and dispassion.

THE CONQUEST OF DESIRE (PAGE 34)
Jīvanmukti-Viveka, chapter 1: "Pramāna-Prakarana." Translation by Georg Feuerstein. This exceptional Sanskrit work was composed by the Vedānta and Yoga master Vidyāranya Tīrtha, who lived in the fourteenth century CE.

THE TWO STREAMS OF THE MIND (PAGE 35)
Yoga-Bhāshya 1.12. Translation by Georg Feuerstein. This is the oldest available Sanskrit commentary on Patanjali's *Yoga-Sūtra* and was probably composed in the fifth century CE. It contains many valuable discussions of the yogic process. The *Yoga-Bhāshya*

is ascribed to the legendary sage Vyāsa, who is also credited with the authorship (or editorship) of the Purānas, the *Mahābhārata*, the *Rāmāyana*, and many other works.

THE BOTTLENECK OF THE MIND (PAGES 36–37)
Adapted from *In Woods of God-Realization: The Complete Works of Swami Rama Tirtha* (Lucknow, India: Rama Tirtha Pratisthan, 1910; 9th ed., 1978), vol. 1, pp. 74–75. Swami Rama Tirtha (1873–1906) was a popular young mathematics professor when, at the beginning of 1901, he renounced the world. He traveled widely around the world, visiting America in 1904, and everywhere imparted the lofty teachings of nondualism. When he was leaving the United States, students who had come to bid him farewell on the ship presented him with typed copies of his lectures in several metal boxes. He thanked them but then joyously surrendered them to the ocean, saying he was not a beast of burden to carry them all the way back to India. Two years later, he drowned while bathing in the Ganges. His talks, which had to be collected from students in many countries, were published posthumously. Hundreds of Swami Rama Tirtha's vivid and inspiring talks are thought to have been lost.

THE POWER OF THOUGHT (PAGE 38)
Maitrī-Upanishad 4.34. Translation by Georg Feuerstein. This Upanishad was probably composed 300–400 BCE.

THE MIND IS THE CAUSE OF BONDAGE AND LIBERATION (PAGE 39)
Amrita-Bindu-Upanishad 1–5. Translation by Georg Feuerstein. This scripture, one of the so-called *Yoga-Upanishads*, was probably composed in the early centuries of the common era.

THE EGO (PAGE 40)
Sri Aurobindo, *A Practical Guide to Integral Yoga: Extracts Compiled from the Writings of Sri Aurobindo and The Mother*

(Pondicherry, India: Sri Aurobindo Ashram, 1955), p. 134. About Sri Aurobindo, see the note to "On the Way to the Divine."

DELETE THE "I"-THOUGHT THROUGH SELF-INQUIRY (PAGES 41–43)

Adapted from *The Teachings of Ramana Maharshi,* ed. Arthur Osborne (York Beach, Me.: Samuel Weiser, 1996), pp. 117–18. Ramana Maharshi (1879–1950), who attained enlightenment spontaneously at the age of sixteen, was one of the twentieth century's greatest sages. He was a living demonstration of the truth of *jnāna-yoga* at the heart of Vedantic nondualism. His fame in the West was primarily due to the advocacy of Paul Brunton (1898–1981), who wrote about his encounter with Ramana Maharshi in *A Search in Secret India* (1934).

THE FIVE HINDRANCES (PAGES 44–45)

Yoga-Sūtra 2.3–16. Translation by Georg Feuerstein. The *Yoga-Sūtra* of Patanjali is the source text of Classical Yoga. It was composed in the period between 300 BCE and 200 CE, with the latter date being more plausible. The theory of the five causes of affliction (*klesha*) is an important aspect of Patanjali's Yoga philosophy. These causes are the primary motor of the unregenerate personality and must be eliminated through the cultivation of wisdom and, more specifically, by means of supraconscious ecstasy (*asamprajnāta-samādhi*).

MENTAL RESTLESSNESS (PAGES 46–48)

Yoga-Vāsishtha 3.112.5–19. Translation by Georg Feuerstein. About this work, see the note to "The Potential of the Body." The epithet Rāghava means "Raghu's descendant" and is often applied to Rāma, who is the spiritual hero of the *Yoga-Vāsishtha*, which is also known as the *Yoga-Vāsishtha-Mahārāmāyana.*

TETHER THE MIND (PAGE 49)

Lallā's *Vākh*, verse 30. Translation by Georg Feuerstein. The mystical sayings (*vākh*, Sanskrit: *vākya*) of Lallā (14th cen. CE) are among Kashmir's magnificent spiritual treasures. Lallā was a great *yoginī* and a master of *kundalinī-yoga*, the Yoga of the serpent power.

BE GRATEFUL TO THE MIND (PAGE 50)
Swami Muktananda, *Play of Consciousness: Chitshakti Vilas* (New York: Harper & Row, 1978), p. 245. Swami Muktananda (1908–83), a great master of *kundalinī-yoga*, initiated thousands of Westerners through direct transmission (*shakti-pāta*).

THE STEED OF THE MIND (PAGE 51)
Translation by V. K. Sethi in *Kabir: The Weaver of God's Name* (Dera Baba Jaimal Singh, India: Radha Soami Satsang Beas, 1984), p. 462. Kabir (1440–1518 CE) was a Muslim who converted to Hinduism under the influence of Rāmānanda and also the Kashmiri poetess-*yoginī* Lallā. The term *sahaj* (Sanskrit: *sahaja*) refers to the "natural" state, that is, the state of perpetual Self-realization.

THREE GREAT OBSTACLES ON THE PATH (PAGES 52–54)
Tripura-Rahasya 20.82–93, 96, 98a. Translation by Georg Feuerstein. The *Tripura-Rahasya*, a Vedānta text inspired by the Tantric Shrī-Vidyā school of South India, was a favorite scripture of the twentieth-century sage Ramana Maharshi. The Goddess uttering the quoted words of wisdom is none other than Tripurā, a form of Devī.

THE FAULT OF INDECISIVENESS (PAGES 55–57)
Yoga-Vāsishtha 6.1.88.1–14; 16. Translation by Georg Feuerstein. About the *Yoga-Vāsishtha*, see the note to "The Potential of the Body."

THE METAPHOR OF THE CHARIOT (PAGE 58)
Katha-Upanishad 1.3.3-8. Translation by Georg Feuerstein. The *Katha-Upanishad*, which belongs perhaps to the sixth or seventh

century BCE, is the first Upanishad to define Yoga and contains many important yogic teachings.

THE NATURE OF KNOWLEDGE (PAGES 59)

Bhagavad-Gītā 13.7–11. Translation by Georg Feuerstein. The *Bhagavad-Gītā*, which is a segment of the *Mahābhārata*, is thought to have been composed around 500 BCE. It is a full-fledged yogic scripture and belongs to the community of Vishnu worshipers, more specifically the devotees of Vishnu's incarnation (*avatāra*) as Krishna. The phrase "Yoga of non-otherness" (*ananya-yoga*) is explained in Shankara's commentary as "ecstasy of nonseparate-ness" (*aprithak-samādhi*), that is, meditative merging with the divine Being, in this case Lord Krishna.

SELF-KNOWLEDGE (PAGE 60)

Adapted from *Talks with Sri Ramana Maharshi*, edited anonymously (1955; reprint, Tiruvannamalai, India: Sri Ramanasramam, 1994), p. 53. About Ramana Maharshi, see the note to "Delete the 'I'-Thought through Self-Inquiry."

YOGA AND WISDOM (PAGE 61)

Trishikhi-Brāhmana-Upanishad 2.19b–22. Translation by Georg Feuerstein. This is a late Upanishad presupposing the full development of *hatha-yoga*. The Sanskrit text of this scripture, like many *hatha-yoga* texts, is defective, though the meaning of each stanza is clear.

THE ULTIMATE FUTILITY OF INTELLECTUAL LEARNING (PAGES 62–63)

Kula-Arnava-Tantra 1.88–98. Translation by Georg Feuerstein. About the *Kula-Arnava-Tantra*, see the note to "The Preciousness of Human Embodiment."

Book Knowledge versus Self-Knowledge (page 64)
Jīvanmukti-Viveka 2. Translation by Georg Feuerstein. About the *Jīvanmukti-Viveka*, see the note to "The Conquest of Desire." Mahādeva is none other than Shiva, the deity of yogis par excellence.

The Need for Discipline (pages 65–66)
Swami Nikhilananda, trans., *The Gospel of Sri Ramakrishna* (New York: Ramakrishna-Vivekananda Center, 1952), p. 363. About Sri Ramakrishna, see the note to "The Fishing-Net of the World."

Making Time for the Divine (page 67)
Complete Works of Ram Chandra (Molena, Ga.: Shri Ram Chandra Mission, 1991), vol. 2, p. 24. Ram Chandra (1899–1983) was the founder of the Shri Ram Chandra Mission, headquartered in Shahjahanpur, in the Indian state of Uttar Pradesh. He taught Sahaj Marg (Sanskrit: *sahaja-mārga*), the path of spontaneity or naturalness, consisting in the constant remembrance of the guru as the Divine itself.

Practice Makes Perfect (pages 68–69)
Yoga-Vāsishtha 3.22.23–31. Translation by Georg Feuerstein. About the *Yoga-Vāsishtha*, see the note to "The Potential of the Body." The Goddess here is Sarasvatī, deity of learning and culture.

Daily Discipline (page 70)
Jīvanmukti-Viveka 3. Translation by Georg Feuerstein. About the *Jīvanmukti-Viveka*, see the note to "The Conquest of Desire."

Asceticism Is Everything (page 71)
Mahābhārata 12.210.15–17. Translation by Georg Feuerstein. About the *Mahābhārata*, see the note to "The Truth about Joy and Sorrow." *Tapas* means both "asceticism" and the "power of

asceticism," the tremendous energy produced by austerities. The Hindu sages have looked upon the work of the creator god, Prajāpati, as a kind of primordial asceticism, which the yogis emulate not to create but to dissolve their own microcosm.

SUCCESS IN YOGA (PAGE 72)
Shiva-Samhitā 3.16ff. Translation by Georg Feuerstein. About the *Shiva-Samhitā*, see the note to "The World Is Illusory."

THE TRUE GURU (PAGE 73)
Adapted from the translation in W. G. Orr, *A Sixteenth Century Indian Mystic* (London and Redhill: Lutterworth Press, 1947), p. 87 (*Gurudeva* 107–11). Dādū (1544–1603 CE), a contemporary of the Muslim emperor Akbar the Great, was initiated by a wandering ascetic at the age of eleven, which led to his renunciation of the world seven years later. His *Bani* (Sayings), composed in Hindi, consist of beautiful poetic hymns extolling the spiritual path of devotion (*bhakti*). Dādū's beliefs and ideas were shaped by both Hinduism and Islam (Sufism). The true teacher or *sad-guru* (from *sat*, "true, real"), not surprisingly, is a frequent focus of the spiritual literature of India.

CHARACTERISTICS OF A SUPERIOR TEACHER (PAGES 74–77)
Kula-Arnava-Tantra 13.67–68, 70–71, 88, 90–91, 104–16, 121–23. Translation by Georg Feuerstein. About the *Kula-Arnava-Tantra*, see the note to "The Preciousness of Human Embodiment." The Sanskrit phrase *kula-nāyikā*, here rendered loosely as "Noble Lady," refers to Shiva's divine spouse, who is the heroine of the Tantric "family" or "flock" (*kula*). The term *pashu*, literally "beast," refers to the ordinary worldling who is ignorant of the path of liberation and is lost in the jungle of conventional existence because he or she is bound by the "bonds" (*pāsha*) of afflictive emotions and erroneous views.

THREE KINDS OF PRECEPTOR (PAGE 78)

Brahma-Vidyā-Upanishad 51b–52. Translation by Georg Feuerstein. This text is grouped among the *Yoga-Upanishads,* which belong to the medieval era. The Sanskrit term *sthāna* refers here to the ultimate Reality, the Self.

CHARACTERISTICS OF A DISCIPLE (PAGES 79–80)

Kula-Arnava-Tantra 13.23–31a. Translation by Georg Feuerstein. About the *Kula-Arnava-Tantra,* see the note to "The Preciousness of Human Embodiment." The phrase *kuleshanī* (from *kula* and *īshanī*), here translated as "Noble Mistress," means literally "Ruler of the Family," the family being the Tantric group of the Kaulas, who created the *Kula-Arnava-Tantra.* The term *āstika,* here rendered as "honoring tradition," refers to a person's faith in the Vedic revelation. This faith or affirmation is known as *āstikya* ("it-is-ness").

FOUR TYPES OF YOGA PRACTITIONERS (PAGES 81–82)

Shiva-Samhitā 5.17–30. Translation by Georg Feuerstein. About the *Shiva-Samhitā,* see the note to "Microcosm and Macrocosm." In Sanskrit, the four types are *mridu-sādhaka* (weak practitioner), *madhyama-sādhaka* (middling practitioner), *adhimātra-sādhaka* (special practitioner), and *adhimātratama-sādhaka* (very special practitioner). *Laya-yoga* is the path of meditative absorption into the Divine preceded by the progressive dissolution of the elements of the mind.

THE NEED FOR INITIATION (PAGE 83)

Mantra-Yoga-Samhitā 5. Translation by Georg Feuerstein. This text is a late Tantric scripture expounding, as the title suggests, the discipline of *mantra-yoga* on the basis of Vedānta. Sacred utterances (*mantra*) are essential to both the Vedic and the Tantric revelation. Initiation is crucial to all forms of Yoga.

KINDS OF INITIATION (PAGES 84–85)

Kula-Arnava-Tantra 14.3–4, 18, 35–39. Translation by Georg Feuerstein. About the *Kula-Arnava-Tantra*, see the note to "The Preciousness of Human Embodiment." Initiation can be external or internal. The most common form of external initiation is by means of ritual. Internal intiation involves a process of penetration (*vedha*) by which the guru enters into the disciple, duplicating his or her own realization. Initiation by means of the alphabet involves the meditative process of projecting the letters of the Sanskrit alphabet upon the disciple's body and then dissolving them in reverse order until the disciple is experiencing the enlightened state directly. Initiation by means of emanation (*kalā*) is a similarly esoteric process, which begins at the soles of the feet and proceeds to the crown of the head. Again the dissolution of the levels of *kalā* creates in the disciple the highest state of consciousness. In the initiation through touch, the teacher triggers the same process by simply touching the disciple, as did Sri Ramakrishna with Swami Vivekananda. In initiation through speech, the guru simply utters a mantra or command. In initiation through vision, the initiatory process is triggered by the teacher's mere gaze. This is also known as *shāmbhavī-dīkshā*. In some cases, it is sufficient for the guru to will the disciple's enlightenment through mere thought.

GOOD COMPANY (PAGE 86)

Tiru-Mandiram 543. Adapted from the translation by B. Natarajan in M. Govindan, ed., *Thirumandiram: A Classic of Yoga and Tantra by Siddhar Thirumoolar* (Montreal: Babaji's Kriya Yoga and Publications, 1993), vol. 1, p. 2–49. About the *Tiru-Mandiram*, see the note to "Cutting through Desire." *Sat-sanga* ("good company") is valued in most yogic schools. According to the *Yoga-Vāsishtha* (2.16.1–2), it increases one's understanding and removes one's ignorance and suffering.

ASSOCIATION WITH HOLY FOLK (PAGES 87–88)
Yoga-Vāsishtha 2.16.1–9. Translation by Georg Feuerstein. About the *Yoga-Vāsishtha*, see the note to "The Potential of the Body." The phrase "association with holy folk" corresponds to the Sanskrit *sādhu-sangama* or *sādhu-samgati* in the quoted passage. A *sādhu* is a "good" or "virtuous" person, whose peaceful presence is helpful to those who come in contact with him.

THE PATH TO LIBERATION (PAGES 89–91)
Mahābhārata 12.266.4–16. Translation by Georg Feuerstein. About the *Mahābhārata*, see the note to "The Truth about Joy and Sorrow."

INTENDING LIBERATION (PAGE 92)
Tripura-Rahasya 20.78–79. Translation by Georg Feuerstein. About the *Tripura-Rahasya*, see the note to "Three Great Obstacles on the Path." Conscious intent (*tatparyatva*) is indeed necessary for any kind of success but especially for the successful completion of one's spiritual discipline. Liberation is realization of one's essential being, the Self (*ātman*).

THINK OF YOURSELF AS IMMORTAL (PAGE 93)
The Complete Works of Swami Vivekananda, 13th reprint (Calcutta: Advaita Ashrama, 1984), vol. 3, p. 130. Swami Vivekananda (1863–1902), the best-known disciple of Sri Ramakrishna, was one of the chief promulgators of Yoga and Vedānta in the West at the turn of the century.

THE CAGED NIGHTINGALE (PAGES 94–95)
Translation in A. J. Alston, *Yoga and the Supreme Bliss: Songs of Enlightenment by Swāmī Rāma Tīrtha* (London: Alston, 1982), pp. 61–62. About Swami Rama Tirtha, see the note to "The Bottleneck of the Mind."

THE INNER TREASURE (PAGES 96–97)
Translation by V. K. Sethi in *Kabir: The Weaver of God's Name* (Dera Baba Jaimal Sing, India: Radha Soami Satsang Beas, 1984), pp. 271–72. About Kabīr, see the note to "The Steed of the Mind."

YOGA AND THE DIVINE LIFE (PAGE 98)
Sri Aurobindo, *A Practical Guide to Integral Yoga* (Pondicherry, India: Sri Aurobindo Ashram, 1976), pp. 67–68. About Sri Aurobindo, see the note to "On the Way to the Divine."

THE FOUNDATION OF FAITH (PAGE 99)
Yoga-Bhāshya 1.20. Translation by Georg Feuerstein. About the *Yoga-Bhāshya*, see the note to "The Two Streams of the Mind." There is an important difference between faith (*shraddhā*) and mere belief. The latter is simply opinion, which can be replaced by other opinions.

THE SUPREME VALUE OF FAITH (PAGE 100)
Bhagavad-Gītā 17.1–4. Translation by Georg Feuerstein. About the *Bhagavad-Gītā*, see the note to "The Nature of Knowledge." All manifestation, whether physical or mental, is understood as an interplay of the three primary qualities (*guna*) of nature (*prakriti*), namely, *sattva, rajas,* and *tamas,* representing the principles of lucidity, dynamism, and inertia respectively.

THE EIGHT LIMBS OF YOGA (PAGES 101–102)
Yoga-Sūtra 2.28–29 with *Yoga-Bhāshya* 2.28–29 (partial rendering). Translation by Georg Feuerstein. About the *Yoga-Sūtra*, see the note to "The Five Hindrances." About the *Yoga-Bhāshya*, see the note to "The Two Streams of the Mind." The *gunas* are the three fundamental qualities of nature, which are radically different from the transcendental Self, or Consciousness. The vision of discernment experientially separates these two basic categories of

existence, leading to the disentanglement of Consciousness from the processes of nature and therefore to liberation. The eight limbs in Sanskrit are *yama, niyama, āsana, prānāyāma, pratyāhāra, dhāranā, dhyāna,* and *samādhi.*

THE EIGHTFOLD PATH (PAGE 103)
Trishiki-Brāhmana-Upanishad 2.28b–32a. Translation by Georg Feuerstein. This Upanishad is one of the medieval *Yoga-Upanishads.* It maps the yogic path against the philosophical backdrop of nondualist Vedānta. This text offers an original interpretation of the eightfold path of Yoga that complements the formal definitions given by Patanjali in his *Yoga-Sūtra* (2.29ff.).

THE MIDDLE PATH (PAGE 104)
Tiru-Mandiram 320, 322. Adapted from the translation by B. Natarajan. M. Govindan, ed. in *Thirumandiram: A Classic of Yoga and Tantra by Siddhar Thirumoolar* (Montreal: Babaji's Kriya Yoga and Publications, 1993), vol. 1, p. 1–35. About the *Tiru-Mandiram*, see the note to "Cutting through Desire." The middle path is none other than the central channel (*sushumnā-nādī*), which is the conduit for the awakened serpent power (*kundalinī-shakti*).

THE PATH IS DIFFICULT (PAGE 105)
Mahābhārata 12.289.50–52. Translation by Georg Feuerstein. About the *Mahābhārata*, see the note to "The Truth about Joy and Sorrow." The path of the knowledgeable brahmins is none other than the path of liberation. Bhāratarshabha is an epithet of Yudhishthira, Arjuna's brother.

SPONTANEITY (PAGE 106)
Translation by Deben Bhattacharya in *Songs of the Bards of Bengal* (New York: Grove Press, 1969), pp. 73–74. Jādubindu, who may have lived in the eighteenth or nineteenth century, was a wan-

dering Bāul who composed numerous songs, which are still sung widely by today's peasants of Bengal. He avowed the path of spontaneity (*sahaja-mārga*). The Bāuls (from Sanskrit *vātula*, meaning "airy" or "mad") are homeless renouncers who travel, either singly or in groups, through Bengal's villages singing, dancing, and playing their simple musical instruments, all the while praising the Divine and the ideal of love (*bhakti*).

FREEDOM IN ACTION (PAGES 107–109)
Bhagavad-Gītā 3.4–9, 19–24; 18.56–57. Translation by Georg Feuerstein. About the *Bhagavad-Gītā*, see the note to "The Nature of Knowledge." *Buddhi-yoga* means literally the "unitive discipline of the higher mind." The *buddhi* is the seat of wisdom. By resorting to it, the yogi gains control over his or her lower personality and increasingly manifests the principle of lucidity (*sattva*) in his or her inner and outer life, thereby drawing ever closer to the Self.

COMMUNE WITH NATURE (PAGE 110)
Swami Sivananda, *Divine Bliss* (Sivanandanagar, India: Divine Life Society, 1964), p. 295. Swami Sivananda (1887–1963) was one of the great modern masters of Yoga. After a successful practice as a physician, he renounced the world in 1923 and founded his own hermitage in 1932. Four years later he established the now famous Divine Life Society. He had numerous disciples, notably Swami Sivananda Radha (a German-born *yoginī*), Swami Satyananda, and Swami Vishnudevananda.

CHANNELING EMOTIONS (PAGE 111)
Swami Sivananda Radha, *Mantras: Words of Power* (Porthill, Idaho: Timeless Books, 1980), p. 23. Swami Sivananda Radha (1911–95), a German-born woman, was a disciple of the famous Swami Sivananda of Rishikesh. She made a significant contribution to translating traditional yogic concepts into modern psychological language and demonstrated that it is possible for contem-

porary Westerners not only to understand but also to tread the ancient path of Yoga.

Base Emotions (pages 112–113)

Shiva-Purāna, Umā-Samhitā 23.20–24, 28. Adapted from the translation in A Board of Scholars, *Ancient Indian Tradition and Mythology,* vol. 3 (Delhi: Motilal Banarsidass, 1969), p. 1547. The *Shiva-Purāna* is counted among the major Purānas, and its scope is truly encyclopedic. It may have been composed around or shortly prior to 1000 CE.

Overcoming Depression (pages 114–115)

Spanda-Kārikā 3.8 with *Spanda-Nirnaya* 3.8 (partial rendering). Translation by Georg Feuerstein. The *Spanda-Kārikā* is attributed to either Vasugupta (the author of the *Shiva-Sūtra*) or to his disciple Kallata (both 9th cen. CE). The *Spanda-Nirnaya* is a scholarly commentary by Kshemarāja (late 10th/early 11th cen. CE).

Give Up Pride (page 116)

Translation by V. K. Sethi in *Kabir: The Weaver of God's Name* (Dera Baba Jaimal Sing, India: Radha Soami Satsang Beas, 1984), p. 596. About Kabīr, see the note to "The Seed of the Mind."

Humility (page 117)

Adapted from the translation by Sardar Sewa Singh in *Sār Bachan*, 7th ed. (Dera Baba Jaimal Singh, India: Radha Soami Satsang Beas, 1978), p. 99 (saying no. 111). The *Sār Bachan* consists of sayings by Swami Maharaj (1818–78), born Seth Shiv Dayal Singh. He was the founder of the Radha Swami sect and first began to teach in 1861 after spending seventeen years in meditation in a dark room. His path is a form of *nāda-yoga*, the Yoga of the inner sound.

Nonviolence (page 118)

Adapted from R. K. Prabhu and U. R. Rao, eds., *The Mind of Mahatma Gandhi* (Ahmedabad: Navajivan Publishing House,

1967), p. 147. First published in the weekly newspaper *Harijan* on June 9, 1946, pp. 172–74. Mohandas Karamchand ("Mahatma") Gandhi (1869–1948) embodied the ideal of self-transcending action, which is at the heart of *karma-yoga*. A lawyer by profession, he opposed the British rule in India by nonviolent means and passive resistance, thus being instrumental in achieving India's political independence.

THE DO'S AND DON'T'S OF SPIRITUAL LIFE (PAGES 119–120)
Bhāgavata-Purāna 7.11.8–12. Translation by Georg Feuerstein. About the *Bhāgavata-Purāna*, see the note to "The Significance of Human Life." The practice of regarding others as oneself (or one's Self) or as divinity is counted as two separate virtues.

LIFE IS A TEST (PAGE 121)
Quoted in M. U. Hatengdi, *Nityananda: The Divine Presence* (Cambridge, Mass.: Rudra Press, 1984), pp. 151–52. Bhagawan Nityananda (1896?–1961), a foundling, attained Self-realization at a very young age and wandered in the Himalayas during his twelfth to sixteenth years. He was made famous in the West by Swami Muktananda.

INNER TRANSFORMATION (PAGE 122)
Anonymous, ed., *Talks with Swami Vivekananda*, reprint (Calcutta: Advaita Ashrama, 1979), pp. 496–97. About Swami Vivekananda, see the note to "Think of Yourself as Immortal."

RIPE AND UNRIPE BEINGS (PAGE 123)
Yoga-Shikhā-Upanishad 1.25–26. Translated by Georg Feuerstein. About this Upanishad, see "The Transmuted Body of the Yogi."

CONTROL OF IMPULSES (PAGE 124)
Mahābhārata 12.288.14–16. Translated by Georg Feuerstein. About the *Mahābhārata*, see the note to "The Truth about Joy and Sorrow." Hamsa ("Swan") is a manifestation of the god Prajāpati,

who assumed the form of a golden swan to wander throughout the cosmos. A *hamsa* is also a particular kind of renouncer, whose home is the entire world.

SILENCE (PAGES 125–126)

Yoga-Vāsishtha 6.1.68.3–9. Translation by Georg Feuerstein. About the *Yoga-Vāsishtha*, see the note to "The Potential of the Body." The five forms of silence in Sanskrit are: *van-mauna* (silence of speech), *aksha-mauna* (silence of the eye), *kāshtha-mauna* (severe silence), *saushupta-mauna* (silence of sleep), and *mano-mauna* (silence of the mind). The last-mentioned involves quieting the mind completely, but only in the condition of living liberation (*jīvan-mukti*) is the mind perfectly transcended. This state corresponds to deep sleep (*sushupti*), though it is marked by the realization of ultimate Awareness, the profound silence of the transcendental Self.

TRUTHFULNESS (PAGES 127–128)

Tiru-Mandiram 2600–04. Adapted from the translation by B. Natarajan in M. Govindan, ed., *Thirumandiram: A Classic of Yoga and Tantra by Siddhar Thirumoolar* (Montreal: Babaji's Kriya Yoga and Publications, 1993), vol. 3, pp. 8–123 and 8–124. About the *Tiru-Mandiram*, see the note to "Cutting through Desire."

THE NATURE OF TRUTH (PAGE 129)

Mahānirvāna-Tantra 4.75–77. Translation by Georg Feuerstein. The *Mahānirvāna-Tantra*, an important Tantric scripture, has been dated between the eleventh and sixteenth centuries CE. The claim made by some scholars that it is a fabrication of the nineteenth century has not been substantiated.

THREE KINDS OF GIVING (PAGE 130)

Bhagavad-Gītā 17.20–22. Translation by Georg Feuerstein. About the *Bhagavad-Gītā*, see the note to "The Nature of Knowledge." *Sattva, rajas,* and *tamas* are the three types of primary energy of nature (*prakriti*), representing the principles of lucidity, dynamism, and inertia respectively. The work of Yoga consists in increasing *sattva.*

SOLITUDE (PAGE 131)
Jīvanmukti-Viveka 1. Translation by Georg Feuerstein. About the *Jīvanmukti-Viveka,* see the note to "The Conquest of Desire."

ALWAYS SERVE OTHERS (PAGE 132)
Swami Sivananda, *Bliss Divine* (Sivanandanagar, India: Divine Life Society, 1964), pp. 293–94. About Swami Sivananda, see the note to "Commune with Nature."

WORSHIP WITH THE BODY (PAGE 133)
Adapted from the translation in W. G. Orr, *A Sixteenth Century Indian Mystic* (London and Redhill: Lutterworth Press, 1947), p. 99 (*Parchā* 230). About Dādū, see the note to "The True Guru."

TRUE WORSHIP (PAGE 134)
Mahānirvāna-Tantra 3.78. Translation by Georg Feuerstein. About the *Mahānirvāna-Tantra,* see the note to "The Nature of Truth."

THE LIBERATING POWER OF DEVOTION (PAGES 135–136)
Bhagavad-Gītā 12.2–8, 14; 18.57–58, 66. Translation by Georg Feuerstein. About the *Bhagavad-Gītā,* see the note to "The Nature of Knowledge."

THE PATH OF DEVOTION (PAGE 137)
Bhakti-Sūtra 5.67–72. Translation by Georg Feuerstein. The *Bhakti-Sūtra* of Nārada is a product of the powerful devotional movement of medieval India. Unlike the more scholarly *Bhakti-*

Sūtra of Shāndilya (600–900 CE) preceding it, this work captures the practical spirit of the movement.

MAD WITH LOVE (PAGE 138)
Adapted from A. J. Alston, *The Devotional Poems of Mīrābāī* (Jawahar Nagar, India: Motilal Banarsidass, 1980), pp. 62–63 (poems 70–71). About Mīrābāī, see the note to "The Time to Realize God Is Now."

LOVE IS THE SELF (PAGE 139)
Adapted from *Talks with Sri Ramana Maharshi,* edited anonymously, 9th ed. (Tiruvannamalai, India: Sri Ramanasramam, 1994), p. 433. About Ramana Maharshi, see the note to "Delete the 'I'-Thought through Self-Inquiry."

THE YOGA OF TEARS (PAGE 140)
Swami Nikhilananda, trans., *The Gospel of Sri Ramakrishna* (New York: Ramakrishna-Vivekananda Center, 1952), p. 182. About Sri Ramakrishna, see the note to "The Fishing-Net of the World."

THE ROAD TO HEAVEN IS THROUGH HELL (PAGE 141)
The Complete Works of Swami Vivekananda, 12th reprint (Calcutta: Advaita Ashrama, 1985), vol. 5, p. 252. About Swami Vivekananda, see the note to "Think of Yourself as Immortal."

HOW TO OVERCOME DEFECTS (PAGE 142)
Manu-Smriti 6.72. Translation by Georg Feuerstein. The *Manu-Smriti* is an ancient work attributed to the lawgiver Manu. In its present form, this scripture belongs to the beginning of the common era, though some of its contents is considerably older. It deals with Yoga in several passages. The "unlordly" (*anīshvara*) qualities mentioned are unbecoming of a yogi because they indicate a lack of self-control.

REAL FASTING (PAGE 143)

Adapted from *Talks with Sri Ramana Maharshi*, edited anonymously (1955; Tiruvannamalai, India: Sri Ramanasramam, 1994), p. 144. About Ramana Maharshi, see the note to "Delete the 'I'-Thought through Self-Inquiry."

THE BEST POSTURE (PAGE 144)

Adapted from *Talks with Sri Ramana Maharshi*, edited anonymously (1955; Tiruvannamalai, India: Sri Ramanasramam, 1994), p. 519. The term *nididhyāsana* denotes "meditation" rather than "one-pointedness," but one-pointedness underlies successful meditation.

THE LIFE FORCE (PAGE 145)

Shiva-Svarodaya 219. Translation by Georg Feuerstein. This is a modern Sanskrit text explaining the fundamentals of *svara-yoga*, the Yoga of the breath (*svara*), which includes a strong divinatory element. The life force, which manifests in the breath, is vitally important to yogis, for it supplies the energetic basis for their work of inner transformation.

BREATH CONTROL (PAGES 146–147)

Yoga-Vāsishtha 5.13.83–92. Translation by Georg Feuerstein. About the *Yoga-Vāsishtha*, see the note to "The Potential of the Body." *Spanda,* or "vibration," is a most important concept in the *Yoga-Vāsishtha,* and one that is especially intriguing to readers familiar with modern cosmology and quantum physics. The phrase "practice of philosophical argument" (*kārana-abhyāsa*) can also be understood as philosophical inquiry into the causes (*kārana*) of things or as yogic practice relative to the sense organs (also called *kārana*).

RESTRAINING THE SENSES (PAGE 148)

Yoga-Shāstra 188–193. Translation by Georg Feuerstein. This is a medieval Sanskrit work attributed to Sage Dattātreya. It focuses on certain locks (*bandha*), seals (*mudrā*), and meditation practices of *hatha-yoga*.

RECITATION ONLY (PAGE 149)
Kula-Arnava-Tantra 15.3–6. Translation by Georg Feuerstein. About the *Kula-Arnava-Tantra*, see the note to "The Preciousness of Human Embodiment." The recitation or repetition of mantras has been a prominent aspect of Yoga since Vedic times and achieved special importance in Tantrism.

SUCCESSFUL MANTRA PRACTICE (PAGE 150)
The Spiritual Teaching of Ramana Maharshi (Boston & London: Shambhala Publications, 1988), p. 56. About Ramana Maharshi, see the note to "Delete the 'I'-Thought through Self-Inquiry."

THE PLEASING INNER SOUND (PAGE 151)
Nāda-Upanishad 42–46a. Translation by Georg Feuerstein. This is one of the *Yoga-Upanishads*. The practice of cultivating the inner sound (*nāda-upāsana*) has been an important feature of *hatha-yoga* from the beginning.

CONCENTRATION (PAGES 152–153)
Sri Aurobindo, *The Synthesis of Yoga*, 4th ed. (Pondicherry, India: Sri Aurobindo Ashram, 1970), pp. 308–09. About Sri Aurobindo, see the note to "On the Way to the Divine."

BE THE OBSERVER (PAGES 154–155)
Maurice Frydman, trans., *I Am That: Conversations with Sri Nisargadatta Maharaj* (Bombay: Chetana, 1976), vol. 2, pp. 145–46. Nisargadatta (1897–1981) was a *bidi* merchant who renounced the world in 1937, but then, cutting short his pilgrimage to the Himalayas, returned to Bombay and his profession to live out the rest of his life in utter simplicity. His wisdom soon attracted people from everywhere. Like Ramana Maharshi, he was a living example

of the truth of nondualism (*advaita*), which is the foundation of the path of wisdom (*jnāna-yoga*).

THE GREATEST WORK (PAGE 156)
Brihad-Āranyaka-Upanishad 1.4.15. Translation by Georg Feuerstein. This Upanishad is thought to be the oldest of this genre (recently dated by some scholars back to 1800 BCE). The meaning of this mystical statement is that because we are the creators of the universe we inhabit, our work is endless. Because of the parallelism between microcosm (human being) and macrocosm (universe), we may look upon ourselves as the world at large and contemplate this great mystery.

TRANSFORM THE WORLD THROUGH MEDITATION (PAGE 157)
Swami Muktananda, *Play of Consciousness: Chitshakti Vilas* (San Francisco: Harper & Row, 1978), p. 14. About Swami Muktananda, see the note to "Be Grateful to the Mind."

OBSTACLES TO MEDITATION (PAGES 158–159)
Yoga-Sūtra 1.30–31 with *Yoga-Bhāshya* 1.30–31. Translation by Georg Feuerstein. About the *Yoga-Sūtra*, see the note to "The Five Hindrances." About the *Yoga-Bhāshya*, see the note to "The Two Streams of the Mind." The word *samādhi,* rendered as "ecstasy," can here stand also for yogic concentration in general. In a deep ecstatic state, the breath can be so unnoticeable that it appears to have stopped altogether. From this vantage point, the breathing of the ordinary worldling seems like a faulty mechanism that interrupts the even flow of consciousness. The close relationship between mind and breath can be seen at work in extreme situations such as terror or anger.

ECSTASY (PAGE 160)
Hatha-Ratna-Avalī 5.1–2. Translation by Georg Feuerstein. The *Hatha-Ratna-Avalī* of Shrīnivāsa Bhatta, an important compen-

dium on *hatha-yoga*, was composed some time in the seventeenth century CE. The two definitions of ecstasy given here follow the metaphysics of Vedānta and differ markedly from the understanding of ecstasy in Patanjali's Yoga, which to all intents and purposes acknowledges a multiplicity of transcendental Selves (*purusha*) and regards liberation as the perfect transcendence of the self.

PATHWAY TO ECSTASY (PAGE 161)

Gheranda-Samhitā 7.1–3. Translation by Georg Feuerstein. The *Gheranda-Samhitā*, a seventeenth-century work, is a classic textbook of *hatha-yoga*. The ten conditions are seeing, hearing, smelling, tasting, touching, sorrow, anger, envy, hatred, and sexual desire. These keep the mind occupied with the finite world and prevent it from realizing the Self. Their suspension coincides with the ecstatic realization of the singular Self.

PSYCHIC POWERS (PAGES 162–163)

Yoga-Shikhā-Upanishad 1.151a–160. About this Upanishad, see the note to "The Transmuted Body of the Yogi." The quality of "otherworldliness" (*alaukika*) refers to the liberated adept's occasional use of paranormal powers, which are also called *gunas* ("qualities" or "virtues") in some texts.

THE SEVEN STAGES OF WISDOM (PAGE 164)

Laghu-Yoga-Vāsishta 6.13.56–60. Translation by Georg Feuerstein. The *Laghu-Yoga-Vāsishta* is an abridgment of the original *Yoga-Vāsishtha*, though some scholars regard the latter to be an expansion of the former. It was composed by Gauda Abhinanda in the ninth century CE. The Sanskrit names of the seven stages are *shubha-icchā, vicāranā, asanga-bhāvanā, vilāpinī, shuddha-samvin-maya-ānanda-rūpā, asamvedanā-rūpā,* and *nirvāna-rūpinī.* "Sameness" stands for the vision of sameness, which is the liberated adept's perfect realization of the same Self in all beings and all beings in the singular Self. The identity of the nine yogis is not clear.

THE SELF IS THE FOUNDATION OF ALL (PAGE 165)

Brihad-Āranyaka-Upanishad 2.4.11–12. Translation by Georg Feuerstein. About this Upanishad, see the note to "The Greatest Work." The Sanskrit word *ātman* means "self" and can refer to "oneself" or "one's self" as well as the single Self of all beings and things, which transcends space and time and which is supreme Being-Awareness-Bliss (*sac-cid-ānanda*, from *sat*, "being"; *cit*, "awareness/consciousness"; and *ānanda*, "bliss"). The teaching about the Self is the great secret revealed in the Upanishads.

FOR THE SAKE OF THE SELF (PAGE 166)

Brihad-Āranyaka-Upanishad 4.5.6. Translation by Georg Feuerstein. About this Upanishad, see the note to "The Greatest Work."

THE IMMORTAL INNER CONTROLLER (PAGES 167–169)

Brihad-Āranyaka-Upanishad 3.7.15–23. Translation by Georg Feuerstein. About this Upanishad, see the note to "The Greatest Work." The key term *antaryāmin* has also been translated as "inner ruler" and "inner guide." The word "guide," however, is too weak for what is intended, because the Self is absolutely in charge of the finite universe and all beings in it. Uddālaka Āruni was one of the great enlightened sages of early Upanishadic times.

THE SERPENT POWER AWAKENS (PAGE 170)

Gopi Krishna, *Kundalini: Path to Higher Consciousness* (New Delhi: Orient Paperback, 1976), pp. 6–7. Gopi Krishna (1903–84) experienced this spontaneous awakening of the serpent power (*kundalinī-shakti*) at the age of thirty-four while meditating. He subsequently wrote many books on the subject and became the world's leading spokesperson for scientific research into this intriguing aspect of the spiritual process. The *kundalinī* is the energy of Consciousness, or Goddess power, and is fundamental to the philosophy and practice of Tantric Yoga and *hatha-yoga*.

THE LONG-HAIRED ASCETIC (PAGES 171–172)

Rig-Veda 10.136. Translation by Georg Feuerstein. This well-known hymn of the archaic *Rig-Veda* is known as the *keshī-sūkta*. The *keshin* is the long-haired ascetic or sage (*muni*) capable of all kinds of feats, but especially the heroic task of bearing or enduring the world by means of his formidable asceticism (*tapas*). He is a friend of the gods Vāyu ("Wind") and Rudra ("Howler"), both of whom are associated with the air and the breath. This hymn (*sūkta*), full of symbolism and mythological allusions, is considered one of the earliest expressions of yogic wisdom. The "unbendable" (*kunamnamā*) mentioned in the last verse has sometimes been equated with the serpent power (*kundalinī-shakti*).

FLOATING IN THE DIVINE (PAGES 173–174)

Adapted from Ram Chandra, *Complete Works of Ram Chandra* (Pacific Grove, Calif.: Shri Ram Chandra Mission, 1989), vol. 1, pp. 374–375. About Ram Chandra, see the note to "Making Time for the Divine."

EMBODIED LIBERATION (PAGES 175–176)

Jnāneshvarī 6.463–71. Adopted from the translation by V. G. Pradhan and H. M. Lambert in *Jnāneshvarī* (London: Allen & Unwin, 1967), vol. 1, pp. 171–72. About the *Jnāneshvarī*, see the note to "Instruction in Happiness." Brahma here is the god Brahma, the creator of the universe. Embodied liberation coincides with the realization of the Absolute (*brahman*), which transcends Brahma and all other deities and their celestial realms.

THE LIBERATED SAGE (PAGES 177–178)

Varāha-Upanishad 4.2.21–30. Translation by Georg Feuerstein. This is one of the so-called *Yoga-Upanishads*, composed in the medieval era. "He who is liberated while still alive" is called *jīvan-mukta* in Sanskrit. His condition is known as *jīvan-mukti*, or "living liberation." The other principal type of liberation is that which coincides with the death of the physical body (and, in fact, the dropping of all bodies or "sheaths"). It is known as *videha-mukti* or "disembodied liberation."

THE SUPREME SWAN (PAGES 179–180)

Paramahamsa-Upanishad 1–3. Translation by Georg Feuerstein. This short Upanishad, consisting of only four sections, describes the type of enlightened adept known as a "supreme swan." The image evoked is that of a being who, completely unattached, roams the world as free as a swan. The "man of the Vedas" (*veda-purusha*) is the adept who not only knows about the Truth intellectually but has become one with it. The Vedas, which are honored as revealed scripture, here symbolize the Truth itself.

HOW DOES THE LIBERATED SAGE BEHAVE? (PAGE 181)

Subāla-Upanishad 13.1. Translation by Georg Feuerstein. This Upanishad, which was composed sometime in the first millennium CE, belongs to what is known as the group of *Sāmānya-Vedānta-Upanishads*. The transcendental state of Aloneness, or *kaivalya*, is the state of liberation, or full recovery of the Self, which, according to Vedānta, is alone (*kevala*) or singular (*eka*). Tree, lotus, and space do not bemoan their destiny. Similarly, the childlike sage does not concern himself with death, for he has realized the immortal Self. Also, anger or wrath (*kopa*), which in a moment can destroy the good merit of lifetimes, does not arise in one who has transcended the ego.

OPEN-EYED ECSTASY (PAGES 182–184)

Tripura-Rahasya 10.1–23a, 36–40. Translation by Georg Feuerstein. About the *Tripura-Rahasya,* see the note to "The Great Obstacles on the Path." Princess Hemalekhā, who is a fully enlightened being, instructs her husband in the significant difference between ordinary ecstasy (*samādhi*) and open-eyed or natural ecstasy (*sahaja-samādhi*). It is passages like this that give the

Tripura-Rahasya its lasting value. Little wonder that a great Self-realized adept like Ramana Maharshi should have favored this work.

LEVELS OF BLISS (PAGES 185–187)

Taittirīya-Upanishad 2.8.1–2.9.1a. Translation by Georg Feuerstein. The *Taittirīya-Upanishad* is among the oldest works of this genre of sacred literature and may have been composed as early as thirty-five centuries ago. Its description of progressively higher levels of ecstatic existence is meant to convey that the bliss of the Absolute exceeds comprehension. Note the distinction between Brahma (the highest deity, the Creator) and *brahman*, the vastly expansive Being who comprises all things, including the god Brahma. "One who is versed in the sacred revelation" (*shrotriya*) is a twice-born member of Hindu society, who has imbibed the values of the Vedic revelation (*shruti*) by carefully listening (*shrotra*) to the recitations and explanations of a teacher.

BLISS BEYOND PAIN (PAGE 188)

R. Powell, *The Wisdom of Sri Nisargadatta Maharaj* (New York: Globe Press Books, 1992), p. 67. About Sri Nisargadatta Maharaj, see the note to "Be the Observer."

I AM FOOD (PAGE 189)

Taittirīya-Upanishad 3.10.5. Translation by Georg Feuerstein. About this Upanishad, see the note to "Levels of Bliss." In the state of ecstatic union, the adept experiences the perfect unity of all things, being both subject ("food eater") and object ("food"). The expression "sound maker" (*shloka-krit*) perhaps refers to the Absolute as the ultimate matrix of the sacred sound OM, which is the source of all manifestation. But it also implies that from this exalted state the adept creates verses (*shloka*) pregnant with spiritual significance.

SALUTATION TO MYSELF! (PAGE 190)
Ashtāvakra-Samhitā 2.11–14. Translation by Georg Feuerstein. The *Ashtāvakra-Samhitā* (or *-Gītā*), a medieval tract, is a popular poetic exposition of nondualism and was a favorite of Swami Vivekananda.

COSMIC CONSCIOUSNESS (PAGES 191–192)
Paramahamsa Yogananda, *Autobiography of a Yogi* (1946; reprint, Nevada City, Calif.: Crystal Clarity, 1993), pp. 143–44. Paramhamsa Yogananda (1893–1952), founder of the Self-Realization Fellowship (headquartered in Los Angeles), was one of the early Yoga adepts who taught in the West.

I AM HE (PAGES 193–194)
Adapted from *In Woods of God-Realization: The Complete Works of Swami Rama Tirtha* (Lucknow, India: Rama Tirtha Pratisthan, 1975), vol. 5, pp. 337–38. About Swami Rama Tirtha, see the note to "The Bottleneck of the Mind." The *turīya*, or "fourth," is the fourth state, transcending waking, dreaming, and sleeping. It is the condition of eternal wakefulness or awareness, which is the Self. Swami Rama Tirtha composed these descriptive lines during the state of ecstasy (*samādhi*), which lasted for several days.

IMMORTALITY (PAGE 195)
Arthur Osborne, *Ramana Maharshi and the Path of Self-Knowledge* (York Beach, Me.: Samuel Weiser, 1970), p. 185. About Ramana Maharshi, see the note to "Delete the 'I'-Thought through Self-Inquiry." Ramana Maharshi spoke these words shortly before the demise of his physical body. For a liberated being, there can be no death, because all identification with the body has ceased.

Recommended Reading

BOOKS

Aurobindo, Sri. *The Synthesis of Yoga*. Pondicherry, India: Sri Aurobindo Ashram, 1976.

An in-depth treatment of the philosophy and practice of Integral Yoga taught by the author, who was one of the great sages of modern India.

Avalon, Arthur (Sir John Woodroffe). *The Serpent Power*. New York: Dover, 1974.

A classic work on traditional *kundalinī-yoga* and *laya-yoga*, giving detailed information about the structures of the subtle body, such as the *cakras* and *nadis*, and including renderings of the *Shat-Cakra-Nirūpana* and the *Pādukā-Pancaka*.

Brunton, Paul. *The Notebooks of Paul Brunton*. 16 vols. Burdett, N.Y.: Larson Publications, 1984–88.

These posthumously published notebooks, a treasure trove for students of Yoga and spirituality in general, complement the author's other books.

Criswell, Eleanor. *How Yoga Works: An Introduction to Somatic Yoga*. Novato, Calif.: Freeperson Press, 1989.

A valuable introduction to a yogic approach favoring body-mind integration and based on the insights of traditional Yoga as well as the author's personal experimentation. It includes a review of yogic processes from a scientific perspective.

Eliade, Mircea. *Yoga: Immortality and Freedom.* Princeton, N.J.: Princeton University Press, 1973.

A comprehensive classic study of Yoga from the broad perspective of the history of religion by a renowned Western scholar who was sympathetic to the tradition.

Feuerstein, Georg. *Introduction to the Bhagavad-Gītā: Its Philosophy and Cultural Setting.* Wheaton, Ill.: Quest Books, 1983.

This book provides the necessary background for studying the *Gītā*, which is not only the earliest available Yoga scripture but also the most widely read.

———. *The Yoga-Sūtra of Patañjali.* Rochester, Vt.: Inner Traditions, 1990.

A word-by-word translation and commentary on Patanjali's aphorisms.

———. *Wholeness or Transcendence? Ancient Lessons for the Emerging Global Civilization.* Burdett, N.Y.: Larson, 1992.

An introductory study of the Yoga tradition from the broad point of view of the evolution of consciousness, following Jean Gebser's model.

———. *The Philosophy of Classical Yoga.* Rochester, Vt.: Inner Traditions, 1996.

This scholarly monograph explores the key philosophical and psychological concepts of Patanjali's Yoga, as they can be derived from a careful study of the *Yoga-Sūtra* itself and only secondarily from the commentarial literature.

———. *The Shambhala Guide to Yoga.* Boston & London: Shambhala Publications, 1996.

A compact introduction to the philosophy, history, and practice of the major branches of the Hindu Yoga tradition.

————. *The Shambhala Encyclopedia of Yoga.* Boston & London: Shambhala Publications, 1997.

The single most comprehensive encyclopedia of Yoga, containing more than two thousand entries and numerous illustrations.

Frawley, D. *Tantric Yoga and the Wisdom Goddesses.* Salt Lake City: Passage Press, 1994.

A popular introduction to Tantrism that is respectful of traditional sources, focusing on the ten wisdom forms of the feminine Divine.

Ghosh, S. *The Original Yoga.* Delhi: Munshiram Manoharlal, 1980.

This volume contains renderings of the *Shiva-Samhitā,* the *Gheranda-Samhitā,* and the *Yoga-Sūtra* together with their transliterated Sanskrit texts.

Govindan, Marshall, ed. *Thirumandiram: A Yoga Classic by Siddhar Thirumoolar.* Translated by B. Natarajan. Montreal: Babaji's Kriya Yoga and Publications, 1993.

A free rendering of what is widely thought to be the greatest Tamil work on Yoga.

Iyengar, B. K. S. *Light on Yoga.* New York: Schocken Books, 1976.

The most comprehensive work on the postures (*āsana*) of *hatha-yoga* by the greatest contemporary exponent of this branch of Yoga. Profusely illustrated.

————. *Light on Pranayama.* New York: Crossroad, 1981.

A companion volume to the above work, equally thorough and useful.

————. *The Tree of Yoga.* Boston: Shambhala Publications, 1989.

Elaborating on the metaphor of a tree, the renowned author furnishes a delightful introduction to the practice of Yoga.

Krishna, Gopi. *Living with Kundalini: The Autobiography of*

Gopi Krishna. Edited by Leslie Shepard. Boston: Shambhala Publications, 1993.

This work, based on the author's personal experience, introduced the concept of the *kundalinī* to wider circles in the West.

Muktananda, Swami. *Play of Consciousness (Chitshakti Vilas).* San Francisco: Harper & Row, 1978.

A first-person account of yogic practice and the higher stages of *kundalinī* awakening by one of the twentieth century's greatest Hindu adepts.

Osborne, Arthur, ed. *The Teachings of Ramana Maharshi.* York Beach, Me.: Samuel Weiser, 1996.

Contains some of the precious conversations between the great sage Ramana Maharshi, who had realized the truth of nonduality, and modern seekers.

Radhakrishnan, Sarvepalli, trans. *The Bhagavadgītā.* London: Routledge & Kegan Paul, 1960.

A widely read translation of the *Gītā*, including the transliterated Sanskrit text and a fine scholarly commentary.

———. *The Principal Upaniṣads* London: Allen & Unwin/New York: Humanities Press, 1974.

Scholarly renderings of eighteen Upanishads, together with the transliterated Sanskrit text, notes, and a valuable introduction to Vedānta.

Sannella, Lee. *The Kundalini Experience.* Lower Lake, Calif.: Integral, 1987.

The author, who pioneered the psychiatric study of the *kundalinī*, provides a highly readable account of the physiological and psychological effects of *kundalinī* awakenings.

Sivananda Radha, Swami. *Hatha Yoga: The Hidden Language.*

Spokane, Wash.: Timeless Books, 1987.

An inspiring practice-oriented exploration of the symbolism underlying a selection of yogic postures (*āsana*).

Subramuniyaswami, S. Satguru. *Dancing with Śiva: Hinduism's Contemporary Catechism*. Concord, Calif.: Himalayan Academy, 1993.

A definitive 1,008-page compendium on the spiritual tradition of Shaivism (the worship of the Divine in the form of Shiva). Profusely illustrated and beautifully produced by the monks of Kauai's Hindu Monastery.

Varenne, Jean. *Yoga and the Hindu Tradition*. Chicago: University of Chicago Press, 1976.

A sound introduction to Yoga, including a rendering of the *Yoga-Darshana-Upanishad*.

Venkatesananda, Swami. *The Concise Yoga Vāsistha*. Albany: State University of New York Press, 1984.

A very readable 400-page abridgment of the voluminous *Yoga-Vāsishtha*.

Vivekananda, Swami. *Raja-Yoga*. New York: Ramakrishna-Vivekananda Center, 1982.

———. *Karma-Yoga and Bhakti-Yoga*. New York: Ramakrishna-Vivekananda Center, 1982.

———. *Jnana-Yoga*. New York: Ramakrishna-Vivekananda Center, 1982.

All of Swami Vivekananda's books are written from the standpoint of Advaita Vedānta. His treatments of *rāja-*, *karma-*, *bhakti-*, and *jnāna-yoga* offer many valuable insights based on his own extensive yogic practice.

Yogananda, Paramahansa. *Autobiography of a Yogi*. 1946.

Reprint. Nevada City, Calif.: Crystal Clarity; or Los Angeles: Self-Realization Fellowship, 1987.

A widely read work filled with unusual characters and yogic miracles experienced by the author during his years of discipleship.

PERIODICALS

Hinduism Today. An excellent monthly magazine for Hindus and students of Hinduism published by the Himalayan Academy and edited by Acharya Palaniswami. $35.00 per year. Address: *Hinduism Today*, 107 Kaholalele Road, Kapaa, HI 96746-9304. Editorial tel.: (808) 822-7032. Subscription tel.: (808) 823-9620 or (800) 850-1008.

Inner Directions. An inspiring and beautifully produced quarterly magazine on spiritual practice, including Hinduism and Yoga, published by the Inner Directions Foundation and edited by Matthew Greenblatt. $18.00 per year. Address: *Inner Directions*, P.O. Box 231486, Encinitas, CA 92023. Tel.: (619) 471-5116.

The Mountain Path. A fine monthly magazine on Ramana Maharshi, Vedānta, and Yoga, published by Sri Ramanasramam and edited by V. Ganesan. $15.00 ($25.00 airmail) per year. Address: *The Mountain Path*, Sri Ramanashramam, P.O. Tiruvannamalai, South India 606 603.

Self-Knowledge. A thoughtful and inspiring quarterly magazine for students of Vedantic *adhyātma-yoga* published by Shanti Sadan. £9.00 per year (non-U.K. subscribers). Address: Shanti Sadan, 29 Chepstow Villas, London W11 3DR, England.

Yoga International. An informative bimonthly magazine published by the Himalayan International Institute and edited by Deborah Willoughby. $15.00 per year. Address: Yoga International, Rural

Route 1, Box 407, Honesdale, PA 18431. Tel.: (717) 253-6241.

Yoga Journal. A wide-ranging bimonthly magazine published by the California Yoga Teachers Association and edited by Rick Fields. $19.97 per year. Editorial offices: 2054 University Avenue, Berkeley, CA 94704. Subscription address: P.O. Box 469018, Escondido, CA 92046-9018. Tel.: (510) 841-9200.

Yoga Life. An inspirational monthly magazine, full of helpful practical advice and local color, produced by the Yoga Jivana Satsangha (established by the late Dr. Swami Gitananda Giri) and edited by Smt. Meenakshi Devi Bhavanani). Address: *Yoga Life,* c/o ICYER, 16-A Mattu Street, Chinnamudaliarchavady, Kottakuppam (via Pondicherry), Tamil Nadu 605 104, India.

Yoga World. A bimonthly international newsletter for Yoga teachers and students, dedicated to authenticity, integrity, and unity, published by the Yoga Research Center and edited by Georg Feuerstein. $18.00 per year. Address: YRC, P.O. Box 1386, Lower Lake, CA 95457. Tel.: (707) 928-9898.

Acknowledgments

I would like to thank the following authors and publishers for permission to reproduce copyrighted materials in the present work.

A. J. Alston (author and publisher) for two excerpts from *The Devotional Poems of Mirabai.*

Shanti Sadan, 29 Chepstow Villas, London WII 3DR, for an excerpt from *Songs of Enlightenment: Poems of Swami Rama Tirtha*, translated by A. J. Alston.

Radha Soami Satsang Beas, P. O. Dera Baba Jaimal Singh, District Amritsar, Punjab, India, for three poems from Dera, for three poems from *Kabir: The Weaver of God's Name* by V. K. Sethi.

Babaji's Kriya Yoga and Publications, Inc., 196 Mountain Road, P. O. Box 90, Eastman, Quebec, Canada JOE 1PO, for adapted excerpts from *Thirumandiram,* translated by B. Natarajan and edited by M. Govindan.

Grove/Atlantic, Inc., 841 Broadway, New York, NY 10003, for the excerpt from *Songs of the Bards of Bengal* by Deben Bhattacharya.

Every effort has been made to contact publishers to obtain their consent for reproducing quotes requiring permission under the existing copyright law. In cases where no response has been forthcoming or where I have been unable to trace the author's or publisher's present address, I would be glad to add a full acknowledgment in future editions of this work as soon as I have been notified.

My heartfelt thanks go to Samuel Bercholz, Peter Turner, Ron Suresha, and the other hardworking behind-the-scenes members of Shambhala Publications, and, as always, to my wife, Trisha, for their part in birthing this book.

About the Editor/Translator

Georg Feuerstein, Ph.D., is an independent scholar trained in Indian philosophy and social anthropology. His interest in India's spirituality was awakened when he was thirteen years old, and he has followed the yogic path in various forms since that time. He is the director of the Yoga Research Center and editor of the Center's *Yoga World* newsletter. He also serves on the board of the Healing Buddha Foundation, Sebastopol, California, and is a contributing editor of *Yoga Journal, Inner Directions,* and *Intuition* magazine. His nearly thirty books include *The Shambhala Guide to Yoga, The Shambhala Encyclopedia of Yoga, Lucid Waking,* and *The Yoga-Sūtra of Patanjali.* Among his forthcoming works are *Shambhala Guide to Tantra* and *The Yoga Tradition.*

If you would like to see his current work, he regularly posts articles on his website at:

http://members.aol.com/yogaresrch/

He may be contacted at:

Georg Feuerstein
Yoga Research Center
P.O. Box 1386
Lower Lake, CA 95457

or by e-mail at:

yogaresrch@aol.com